The Vitamin Murders

The Vitamin Murders

Who Killed Healthy Eating in Britain?

James Fergusson

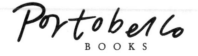

Published by Portobello Books Ltd 2007

Portobello Books Ltd
Eardley House
4 Uxbridge Street
Notting Hill Gate
London W8 7SY, UK

A CIP catalogue record is available form the British Library

9 8 7 6 5 4 3 2 1

13-digit ISBN 978 1 84627 014 7

www.portobellobooks.com

Text designed by Richard Marston
Maps designed by Emily Faccini

Typeset in Palatino by Avon DataSet Ltd,
Bidford on Avon, Warwickshire

Printed by Creative Print and Design, Wales

For Amelia

Contents

Prologue

We found the Drummond family grave entirely by chance. Melissa and I, on holiday in Provence with my parents, had borrowed the family Volvo for the day and gone exploring with no particular itinerary along the upper Durance valley. We spent most of the morning wandering the medieval walled town of Manosque, visiting a dull museum dedicated to the writer Jean Giono, and a church containing an eleventh-century statue of the Black Madonna. By the time we reached Forcalquier, however, that town's cultural highlight, the twelfth-century Notre-Dame du Bourguet, was unaccountably locked.

It was the middle of August and fast becoming too hot for tourism. The restaurants in the shady square below the church looked more tempting than ever. Melissa, ever the professional foodie, had already inspected the menu of one of them while I was parking the car. It was called the *Lapin Tant Pis*, and she came back grinning with the news that it specialized in lamb with lavender honey, and aubergine and cardamom confit. But it was still just too early for lunch, and the tables and chairs arranged beneath the ancient plane trees were all unoccupied.

'Better do something else, I suppose,' said Melissa, peering at a guidebook. 'The "campo santo" might be worth a look. It's a cemetery – nineteenth century. A listed monument. Famous for its yew topiary work.'

A short traipse to the town's edge brought us to a gate in a high perimeter wall. Once inside we could see immediately why the cemetery was considered so special. The place was immense. We were standing at the top of a steep staircase off which led a maze of terraced gardens, each of them fenced in by a thick yew hedge, twelve or more feet high. Deep alcoves cut into the hedges brought to mind a series of interlocking green cloisters. Beyond the cemetery lay miles of lavender fields and olive groves, the landscape dotted with farmhouses of pale yellow stone that shone in the blazing sun; in the hazy distance beyond, the grey foothills of the Alps blended into the sky.

We plunged downwards, struck off at random into one of the gardens, and quickly lost ourselves in the labyrinthine interior. A hole in the hedge led to another garden, and another. There were other staircases to explore, too. It was as though we had stepped into a design by M. C. Escher. Each garden was centred on a manicured lawn with the dead tightly packed around the edge like shrubs in a flowerbed, the graves interspersed with overblown statuary in the loftiest Catholic sepulchral manner. Around every corner lay another ponderous urn in black marble or a hefty angel in lichen-mottled basalt.

The Drummonds' resting place was on the far side of the last garden at the bottom of the main staircase. Our attention was drawn to it by a middle-aged woman with bleached blonde hair – the only other person that we had so far seen in this wonderland. Her back was turned towards us, and at first we assumed she was a mourner, but there was something about her posture, or maybe the brightness of her clothes, that suggested some other reason for her presence here.

Melissa hung back, but I sidled up next to the stranger, curious to see what she was looking at. There were three wooden crosses planted in deep gravel retained by a border of variegated granite. It looked a bit like a giant cat litter box. The names on the crosses were clearly Anglo-Saxon, although spelled without apology in the French way, with one 'm': 'Drumond Anne' on the left, 'Drumond Jack' on the right, and in between, beneath a thick stone slab, 'Drumond Elisabeth'. The plot was peppered with tawdry pieces of ceramic. There was a Bible balanced on its spine, two overlapping lozenges bearing a bas-relief dove, and several faded rings of roses. There were real roses, too: fresh ones still in their cellophane, carefully arranged in flower-holders. The grave bore no dates but it was well weathered. The Drummonds could not have died recently, but they had evidently not been forgotten. 'They were lovely and pleasant in their lives,' the English epitaph read. 'In their death they were not divided.'

I looked again at the blonde woman next to me. She was clutching a digital camera and an oversized purple handbag, and her polyester trousers were a little too short.

'Are you family?' she said suddenly.

'Er, no. But I am an *Anglais*.'

She smiled sombrely.

'That's good. What do you think of the flowers?'

'Mm, lovely,' I replied, and she nodded her satisfaction, as though doing the right thing by the Drummonds were a matter of national honour. 'Madame, I'm sorry to ask, but – who were these people?'

'You don't know?'

'I've never heard of them.'

'But they're very famous – the victims of the most famous murder in France!'

'Murdered? When?'

'Oh, fifty years ago at least. But they're still talking about it on television.'

'Why?'

'Because . . . because it was all a conspiracy. The government was involved, and the KGB. Jack Drummond was a distinguished English scientist, but also a secret agent. And then a farmer called Dominici was framed for the murders . . . I can't believe you don't know all this.'

'Who are the other two?'

'That's his wife, Anne, and their daughter Elisabeth in the middle. They were on holiday, camping by their car at the side of a road not far from here. A place called Lurs. Jack and Anne were shot at close range, but the poor little one . . .'

She dropped her voice here, and leant towards me conspiratorially.

'The poor little one was clubbed to death with the empty rifle. She tried to run away, but they caught her and hit her so hard that the stock of the gun snapped . . . the doctor who examined her skull said it was like handling a bag of nuts. The poor thing was only ten.'

'My God.'

'Yes: a horrible death. Horrible.'

She looked back at the girl's grave with such sorrow that she seemed about to cry, but she pulled herself together at the last moment.

'I was speaking this morning to a man in the village at Lurs,' she went on. 'He told me that the Drummonds aren't actually buried here. Their family couldn't stand for it and secretly had their bones moved back to England. Do you think it's true?'

'I . . . I've no idea. I suppose it's possible.'

'I've read all the books, you know,' she said, cocking her head to one side. 'It wouldn't surprise me if the bones had been moved. Not at all.'

'Are there many books about the murders? Which one would you recommend?'

'There was one by that television journalist . . . oh, I can't remember his name. Anyway, it was very convincing. You should read it.'

'I'm sure I will.'

'Well, if you'll excuse me . . . I must take some photographs. My husband and children in Lyons will want to see this. I was worried that it might seem disrespectful, but you don't mind, do you?'

'Not at all.'

Melissa had come alongside with a quizzical look, and now I gestured to her that we should leave.

'What was all that about?' she said when we were out of earshot.

We walked on through the topiary, and I repeated what I had been told.

'Yuk,' she said, more affected than I had anticipated. 'How could anyone do that to a ten-year-old girl? It's like something out of a slasher movie.'

'Maybe it was intended as a political warning of some sort. If, for instance, this Drummond character really was a secret agent.'

'Or maybe the killer was driven insane by the sun, like Meursault. God, it's hot today.' Melissa had just finished reading Albert Camus' *L'Étranger*, a holiday book chosen because its author had once lived in this region (and indeed was buried just down the valley, at Lourmarin). We had been discussing the book's central scene in the car on the way to Forcalquier, in which the anti-hero, Meursault, his head turned by the scorching Mediterranean sun, shoots dead an Arab on an Algerian beach. Melissa was certainly right about today's heat, which, improbably, was still intensifying. We squinted despite our sunglasses in the light bouncing off the ground; the gravel on the path ahead was so hot that it was uncomfortable even through the soles of our shoes. It wasn't hard to see how one might not be wholly responsible for the consequences of one's actions during *les grandes chaleurs*, as the French called the dog days of August, because the temperature was truly brain-fuddling. Even the simple act of walking demanded an unlikely amount of effort. The path along the bottom of the cemetery seemed much longer than we knew it to be from our earlier overview of it. Our conversation began to dwindle, until the only sound was the remorseless buzz of cicadas and the rhythmic crunch of our footsteps.

As we approached the far end of the cemetery, however, we discerned a new noise, a low mechanical roaring sound that blended in with the cicadas. The source was revealed as we rounded a corner: a ground-keeper, chasing an arc of twigs and sweet papers along the path before him with a leaf-blower. He switched his machine off when he heard our shouted *saluts*, and removed his ear-defenders with a toothless grin.

'We've been to see the Drummonds,' I began.

The ground-keeper nodded and said nothing.

'I expect a lot of people come to see them here?'

'Oh yes. Many.'

'How many?'

'Thirty or forty, most days.'

'Thirty or forty a day!'

'Of course – why not?' he replied. 'Ils sont des vedettes – they are stars!'

I pointed at the leaf-blower and congratulated him on the condition of his cemetery: it looked a lot of work, keeping a place this size in order.

'It is,' he replied. 'I work here all by myself, and the weeding has to be done by hand.'

'Why don't you use weed-killer?'

'I can't. Weed-killer would kill all the yew trees.'

As we laboured back up a staircase to the entrance gate we passed an old *cabanon*, one of the beehive-like stone constructions that, according to our guidebook, the Forcalquier region was famous for. This one seemed to be in use as the ground-keeper's shed. A low door in its side had been left temptingly ajar; out of sight down the hill, the leaf-blower had started up again. We looked left, and right, and ducked beneath the lintel. It was dark and cool inside, and smelled deliciously of old mown grass and two-stroke engine oil. Rakes and shears were visible in the spidery gloom, neatly arranged on hooks above a half-repaired chainsaw on a battered workbench. I also noticed that the ground-keeper's assertion that he didn't use weed-killer wasn't true. On a shelf at the back were several plastic canisters of a liquid chemical called Elegia: 'Désherbant total pour la destruction des mauvaises herbes annuelles', the label read.

It sounded powerful: a kind of Final Solution for all annual weeds. It was an odd thing for the ground-keeper to have lied about.

'Perhaps he only uses it on the non-yew tree bits,' Melissa said, cocking her ear towards the door. 'By the way – can you still hear him?'

We looked at each other, holding our breath. The cicadas outside, though muffled by the stone walls of the *cabanon*, were still perfectly audible. The leaf-blower's faint undertone, on the other hand, had unquestionably stopped. We scrambled through the entrance as though something evil was chasing us. But there was no ground-keeper outside to confront us, nor any other living soul to be seen. We giggled like guilty schoolchildren as we continued up the hill, climbing faster than before, our pace adrenalized by the thrill of almost being caught. The *Lapin Tant Pis*, furthermore, would be open now. It was time for another ill-deserved, irresistible French lunch.

Chapter 1

The Golden Age of Nutrition

'The opening of the 20th century saw malnutrition more rife in England than it had been since the great dearths of medieval and Tudor times. Yet apart from a handful of social workers there were few who showed any real concern at the terrible distress in the working-class districts. Sometimes it comes as a rude shock to realize how great is the inertia to be overcome before the public conscience can be awakened in the matter of social reforms.'

The Englishman's Food by J. C. Drummond and Anne Wilbraham (1939)

It wasn't until the holiday was over and we were back in London that I got around to looking into the killings in more detail. The tourist lady from Lyons had not exaggerated: the triple crime of August 1952 was gruesome. Despite the massive injuries to her cranium, little Elisabeth – or Elizabeth, as she was actually christened – had taken several hours to die. The fact that she was Jack and Anne's only child somehow made it worse; it was as though she were the victim of some evil scheme to extinguish the family line. But on later reflection, the savagery with which she had been finished off eclipsed this dynastic tragedy. The determined ruthlessness of it defied normal understanding. It was evident from the newspapers of the time that the murders had been widely reported. Public opinion on both sides of the Channel was immediately electrified. Camping holidays in France had become increasingly popular among British families in the austere years of the early 1950s. Clement Attlee's

Labour government, terrified of losing control of domestic money supply, had restricted the amount that Britons could take abroad to £50 per person per year (and to £35 per child under twelve), which ruled out flying long distances or travelling anywhere very far on holiday. For a generation forced into parsimony, France was one of the few choices available – a choice that was particularly attractive to motorists, who were allotted an additional £25 if they were taking their own car across the Channel. The murders therefore sent a frisson through tens of thousands of would-be British holiday-makers. It had not occurred to people that camping out in the idyllic French countryside might actually be dangerous. A friend of my father's, a man of about seventy, told me he remembered the murders well because the news prompted his family to alter their French holiday plans at the last minute. There must have been many another British family who took a similar decision that summer. Yet there was more to the story than tabloid sensationalism – a lot more.

Who killed the Drummonds, and why? Those questions had gripped the French for more than half a century. A lengthy police investigation eventually led to the arrest and conviction of one Gaston Dominici, an aged peasant farmer next to whose land the Drummonds had camped. But both the investigation and the subsequent trial were badly botched, and Dominici's guilt was never satisfactorily proved. His death sentence was commuted to life in prison. Shortly before his natural death he was quietly released, on health grounds, on the orders of President de Gaulle himself.

Since then a small industry of conspiracy theories had grown up around 'l'affaire Dominici'. It was probably the most famous French murder mystery of the twentieth century, with a bibliography to rival the Dreyfus Affair's for size. Dozens of books and hundreds of articles had been published over the years. Dedicated pundits had forged entire careers for themselves. There was even a specialist website with an online chatroom where members of the public were invited to advance their own hypotheses. France remained fascinated by it. The journalist

Jean Laborde, who covered the murder trial and later wrote a book about it, noted the unusual mesmerizing quality of the Dominici Affair more than thirty years ago: 'Pour quiconque s'en occupe,' he observed, 'l'affaire Dominici se transforme en obsession.' No-one, it seemed, was more obsessed than Gaston's grandson Alain. A babe-in-arms at the time of the murders, he had spent his entire adult life campaigning for a posthumous state pardon for his grandfather, movingly determined to clear his family name.

The conspiracy theory alluded to by the lady in the cemetery was probably the most popular. It was also one of the most fantastic. Its main exponent was an investigative journalist called William Reymond – a Frenchman, despite the name – who published a book in 1997 in which he accused Drummond of being a British secret agent. Among other things he suggested that the family were not murdered by Gaston Dominici at all, but assassinated by a KGB hit squad. Moscow's motive, according to Reymond, was that Drummond was involved in Operation Paperclip, the Anglo-American attempt to lure away the Eastern Bloc's best scientists in the years immediately after World War Two. In collaboration with Alain Dominici, Reymond published a further book in 2003 that was designed to coincide with a two-part TF1 television dramatization of his improbable theory. The show, which cost £4.5m to make and starred the actor Michel Serrault, a household name in France, was a full-blown media *événement*. It attracted 12 million viewers on both nights – one in five of the population. The makers claimed it was the most watched French television programme of the year.

I was intrigued by France's fascination with the murders, but that was not what most attracted me to the Drummond story. To the French, the fact that Drummond was a distinguished scientist – an upstanding English knight whose work had been honoured by the University of Paris, no less – merely added piquancy to a scintillating murder mystery, but I soon discovered that he was more interesting than that. He wasn't any old scientist, but a food scientist. And not just any food scientist, either, but a noted pioneer in the field of human nutrition. Before Drummond, vitamins A, B and C were called fat-soluble A, water-soluble B and anti-scorbutic factor, and the word 'vitamin' was spelled 'vitamine'. Dropping the ultimate 'e' was his idea, as was the now globally recognized system of vitamin classification.

I had been thinking about food scientists recently – ever since spotting a particular advertisement on the side of a bus in our local high street. It was for Yeo Valley Organic, the Somerset dairy operation, and it depicted a puppet in a white coat with sticking-out hair and mad, swirling green eyes, above the caption 'FOOD SCIENTISTS Я NOT US'. The puppet reminded me a little of Judge Doom in *Who Framed Roger Rabbit?*, the psychotic half-human bent on destroying all cartoon life with his evil chemical 'dip'. The contrast with Jack Drummond, a revered philanthropist knighted for his services to the nation, could hardly have been greater. The good reputation of food scientists had undergone the most dramatic reversal. I described the advertisement later to Melissa. As a specialist supplier of independent restaurants and a former restaurant manager, she was naturally interested in such things.

'The food scientists have got no-one but themselves to blame,' she said. 'They're the ones who invented Turkey Twizzlers, after all.'

Earlier in the week we had cheered on Jamie Oliver, the celebrity TV chef, as he tried to overhaul the repulsive 37p-a-head menu of a state school canteen in Greenwich. The Turkey Twizzler, a fatty, spiral-shaped piece of mechanically rendered turkey meat, was already nationally infamous, an emblem of all that was wrong with industrialized school food. Melissa had met Oliver once. His Shoreditch restaurant, Fifteen, was among those supplied by her company. Now he had made a television series called *Jamie's School Dinners* with the intention of proving that it was possible to mass-produce edible and healthy meals for only slightly more money. The series was well on the way to embarrassing the government into taking official action. (It was later announced that chocolates, crisps and fizzy drinks were to be banned from school vending machines in favour of muffins, yoghurt and fruit.) Jamie Oliver, in short, was a latter-day Jack Drummond. The mantle of philanthropy had been passed on. The murder victim was the grand-daddy of campaigning nutritionists, a man who dedicated much of his life to the eradication of malnutrition in the inner cities. The spectacle of angry parents thrusting bags of chips through the railings of a Greenwich school playground, convinced that the TV chef temporarily inside the building wasn't feeding their offspring properly, would have dismayed him – and he had been a schoolboy in Greenwich himself once, one hundred years before.

In February 1940, a month after the introduction of rationing, the coiner of the word 'vitamin' was appointed Chief Scientific Adviser to the Ministry of Food, where he did more than perhaps any other single individual to ensure that island Britain survived the Nazi U-boat blockade without starving. In fact the health of the British nation, schoolchildren included, was not just maintained during World War Two but *improved*. The American Public Health Association, which cited Drummond for a prestigious Lasker Award after the war, reported that 'the rates of infantile, neo-natal and maternal mortality and still births all reached the lowest levels in the history of the country. The incidence of anaemia and dental caries declined, the rate of growth of schoolchildren improved, progress was made in the control of tuberculosis, and the general state of nutrition of the population as a whole was up to or an improvement upon pre-war standards.' The Americans might also have mentioned that rickets, a painful bone condition caused by vitamin D deficiency, was wiped out in the inner cities. Indeed, the incidence of almost every diet-related illness was lower than it had ever been. As they said in New York, Drummond's rigorously scientific organization of Britain's wartime diet was 'one of the greatest demonstrations in public health administration that the world has ever seen'. He was a genuine Home Front hero.

His achievement was all the more extraordinary given that until the war he was just another academic, a professor of biochemistry at University College London and almost unknown beyond the rarefied circles in which he habitually moved. The turning point in his career was the publication in 1939 of his only book, *The Englishman's Food: A History of Five Centuries of English Diet*. The critical acclaim this work received brought him to the attention of Lord Woolton, the newly appointed Minister of Food; a senior advisory job soon followed.

I ordered a copy from an online second-hand bookshop. The green-bound volume that arrived was a tatty second impression from early 1940. The pages were foxed and thumbed, the dust-jacket was missing, and the frontispiece bore a library stamp from Cambridge University's Anatomy Department. Drummond did not write the book alone but collaborated with one Anne Wilbraham. A previous reader had carefully bracketed the two names on the title-page with a pencil, and noted: 'murdered Aug. 5, 1952'. Drummond's co-author, I realized for the first time, was his unfortunate wife-to-be. I later found out that she was his research assistant at UCL, and thirteen years his junior. The pair had only married in 1940. *The Englishman's Food* was no ordinary book, therefore, but a monument to a romance – indeed to an illicit romance, since Drummond had been married for twenty-four years to Mabel Straw, a schoolmaster's daughter whom he had met in his student days. Their childless marriage broke up in 1939, the split precipitated by the affair with Anne.

The title sounded dry, but the book turned out to be a highly readable blend of social history and biochemistry. It was even funny in places. Drummond had a natural gift for explaining complicated facts simply. It was obvious not only that he knew a great deal about nutrition, but also that he was passionate about his subject. *The Englishman's Food* was a labour of love in more ways than one. I found myself unexpectedly gripped by an account of a fearless young Glaswegian called William Stark, to whom the book was dedicated. Stark, who was born in 1740, experimented on himself in a bid to identify the causes of scurvy. He began by putting himself on a diet of bread and water with an occasional allowance of sugar. Unsurprisingly, after ten weeks he was complaining of bleeding gums and sore nostrils – the first signs of the disorder. He recovered his health with half a pint of blackcurrants, but after several similar experiments, the last of which involved eating nothing but honey puddings and Cheshire cheese, his scurvy turned chronic. 'A true martyr to science', he died of an intestinal disorder on 23 February 1770, aged twenty-nine.

There was much else of interest. I discovered, for instance, what a short-term prison inmate could expect to eat in 1864 – 1600 calories and 97 grams of protein a day – and how his diet compared to that of a fifteenth-century peasant. (The peasant ate twice as much.) The section on infant-feeding in the eighteenth century was just as intriguing. In 1740 the Royal College of Physicians were divided on whether it was better for orphaned babies to be farmed out to wet-nurses or fed cow's milk via a contraption called a 'bubby-pot' that used the finger of a glove as a teat. The answer apparently depended on whether or not the wet-nurse had a gin habit.

Yet the book was more than a collection of dietary curiosities. Its historical perspective illustrated quite how much and how often our eating habits had changed. No-one had attempted such a wide-ranging survey of the national diet before. The demise of the traditional English breakfast was a case in point. For centuries this important meal consisted not of bacon and eggs (which was an invention of the hotel trade in the nineteenth century, and was in any case more Scottish than English), but of herrings and porridge. By the time Drummond wrote his book, this ideal combination of essential fatty acids was already being supplanted by what Britons currently eat in the mornings: breakfast cereal, in league with the sugar industry.

Modern food producers, Melissa observed, were always claiming that they were powerless to alter people's eating habits, and that they were only giving the public what they wanted. *The Englishman's Food* suggested that the opposite was the case. Drummond showed that the population had never been canny about what was good for them, and so had always been susceptible to advertising and suggestion. Thanks to television, they still were – particularly children. What other explanation could there be for a product called *Bart Simpson's Eat My Shorts* – described by the manufacturers, Kellogg's, as 'a frosted golden-syrup-flavored multi-grain cereal shaped like Bart's shorts'? The public wanted what the public got, not the other way round.

It was obvious that Drummond was genuinely angry about the legacy of the Industrial Revolution. Standards of public nutrition had plummeted in the nineteenth century as agricultural workers abandoned the land for the factories in the cities. For the author, the effects of this shift were more than just a subject for academic study – they were a real and emotive social problem. It seemed genuinely to offend him that rickets was still prevalent among the poorest urban classes despite all the progress of modern science.

I finished the book and paid a visit to the Royal Society, the prestigious scientific academy on Carlton House Terrace to which Drummond was elected a Fellow in 1944. The archive section contained a collection of obituaries, from which I learned that Drummond's experience of inner-city deprivation was almost certainly gained at first hand, for his origins were nothing if not humble. He was born in Kennington in south London on 12 January 1891, the son of Major John Drummond of the Royal Horse Artillery, the son of another soldier, a sergeant in the same regiment. John died of bronchitis three months after Jack's birth, aged fifty-five. There was no immediate explanation of what happened to his mother, Gertrude; but for whatever reason, Jack was adopted and raised by John's sister, Maria Spinks, who lived in nearby Charlton. Life in the elderly Spinks household cannot have been fun for the solitary boy. Maria was a strict nonconformist who insisted on Jack's accompanying her to chapel; her husband, George, a retired captain quartermaster who had seen action in the Crimea, was keen on gardening.

Drummond's interest in nutrition dated from his early twenties. After attending schools in Greenwich and the Strand, he graduated in 1912 in chemistry with a First from East London College (now Queen Mary, University of London). In 1914 he was appointed an assistant at the Cancer Hospital Research Institute. Here he came under the influence of one Casimir Funk, whose curious experiments with pigeons and the nutritive value of rice polishings led ultimately to the discovery of vitamin B. It was Dr Funk who first used the word 'vitamine' to describe this and other 'accessory food factors', which he defined as essential to all normal animal growth, in 1912; Drummond proposed dropping the terminal 'e' in 1920 for simplicity's sake. Funk encouraged Drummond to think for the first time about the relationship between diet and disease. The foundations were laid for a lifetime's study of human nutrition.

Most of Drummond's colleagues went off to the trenches during World War One, but the Institute stayed open, and Drummond, whose weak heart excluded him from military service, remained. The authorities recognized the contribution the Institute had to make to the war effort, and Drummond duly played his part. Food rationing was not introduced until late in the war, in February 1918, even though shortages had already caused severe malnutrition among many poor urban communities by the winter of 1916 – including those parts of London where Drummond grew up. When he was invited by the Food (War) Committee of the Royal Society to measure the vitamin content of margarine and other butter substitutes therefore, he threw himself into the project with an enthusiasm that was heartfelt.

By 1918 he was already an acknowledged expert on nutrition. In 1922, at the young age of thirty-one, he was appointed to UCL's newly created Chair of Biochemistry, where he remained until 1939. The department that he built up was small, but its influence on the development of the new academic field of biochemistry was out of all proportion to its size.

Nine of his former pupils or colleagues went on to occupy university chairs elsewhere, a record unmatched by any other British school of biochemistry.

His obituaries agreed that he was an inspired teacher and an outstanding lecturer. He brought a special brand of 'breezy vitality and energy' to his work for which he had an 'almost childish exuberance and enthusiasm'. He was like 'human quicksilver', according to one colleague, because of the way he 'darted from one thing to another and from one problem to another'. He was also a genuine inspiration to his undergraduates, who adored him. Some tried to emulate his peculiar communicator's gift. One of his protégés was Magnus Pyke, the arm-waving star of the 1970s TV science show *Don't Just Sit There*, which I used to watch as a schoolboy.

In some respects Drummond's mind was not well suited to the grind of laboratory work. Detail bored him: he preferred a broader canvas, and to think about the practical application of the emerging knowledge of vitamins and nutrition. Increasingly through the 1930s he gave the appearance of a scientist in a hurry – a man who knew he was leading a revolution in biochemical knowledge, and who believed passionately in the importance of disseminating that knowledge to the public. Official interest in the question of public nutrition was greatly boosted by concerns over the effects of the Depression of the 1930s. A British Medical Association report in 1936 showed that a 'completely adequate healthy diet' was beyond the economic reach of half the British population. But it was the eve-of-war timing of the publication of *The Englishman's Food* that really launched Drummond, because the book demonstrated brilliantly that malnutrition was not just a social issue but also a pressing military one.

Drummond explained how, in 1902, the army's Inspector of Recruiting reported that he was having trouble finding enough men with the necessary physique for service in the Boer War. Nationally, nearly 40 per cent of would-be recruits were rejected; in some places the rate was 60 per cent. The main reasons given were bad teeth, poor sight or hearing, 'heart affections' and deformities. 'So serious was the shortage,' Drummond wrote, 'that it was found necessary to reduce the minimum height for recruits for the infantry to 5 ft; it had already, in 1883, been lowered from 5 ft 6 in to 5 ft 3 in.'

Poor nutrition could also directly affect the performance of troops in the field. In 1918, for instance, an exceptionally large number of German infantrymen fractured their arms while throwing stick bombs. Drummond attributed this to defects in the bone caused by a deficiency of vitamins A and D. The British army, too, had had their share of nutritive disasters. He told the story of General Townsend's expeditionary force in Iraq in 1916, which capitulated at Kut for want of food. This tragedy was 'hastened by the ravages of scurvy and beri-beri among the men' – diseases that could have been alleviated by an airdrop of just a small amount of vitamins B1 and C. Drummond commented: 'There is cruel irony in the fact that an aeroplane did drop a packet to bring relief to the starving garrison; it contained opium to deaden the pangs of hunger.' The book's message could not have been clearer or more timely.

When war was declared in 1939, the British government already knew how difficult it was going to be to feed the home population. The country's dependence on food imports had grown steadily since the Industrial Revolution. The purpose of the British Empire was trade. Importing food made economic sense, but from a military viewpoint it was also the Empire's Achilles' heel. By 1939, Britain was dependent on imports for almost two-thirds of its food supply, above all on wheat from the US and Canada. German attacks on supply ships in the Atlantic had forced David Lloyd George's government to introduce rationing in 1918. The U-boat campaign this time around was even more devastating. At the height of it in 1940, Hitler's submariners destroyed 2.6 million tons of merchant shipping. Winston Churchill later wrote that it was the only time that he ever contemplated surrender. But at least his government had not been taken by surprise. A Ministry of Food had already been established with the monumental task of ensuring that Britain did not starve. Rationing was introduced as the war began, not at the end as before.

Frederick Marquis, Lord Woolton, the Minister of Food, was an ex-managing director of a northern chain store with a pronounced philanthropic bent. He was also a shrewd administrator with first-hand experience of the difficulties of high-volume provision: for a brief period after World War One he had been Controller of Civilian Boot Production. He understood that rationing alone would not be enough to save the Home Front from collapse, and fully appreciated the need for expert advice. According to Magnus Pyke, who followed his mentor Drummond from UCL to the Ministry, one of the first questions that 'Freddie' asked when he was appointed in early 1940 was, 'Where are my scientific advisers?' Brought before the Minister, Drummond produced a plan for the distribution of food based on 'sound nutritional principles', and presented Woolton with a complimentary copy of *The Englishman's Food* for good measure. 'I was more fortunate than any man deserved to be in finding him,' Woolton later remarked.

It was the moment Drummond might have been waiting for all his life. Advising the Ministry was more than just an interesting job to him. From the start he regarded rationing as the perfect opportunity to attack what he called 'dietetic ignorance' and recognized early on that, if successful, he would be able not just to maintain but to improve the nation's health. He was the brains behind an extraordinary campaign of public dietary education that was ultimately more effective than even he had hoped. Rationing combined with sound dietary advice introduced more protein and vitamins to the diet of the poorest in society, while the better off were obliged to cut their consumption of meat, fats, sugar and eggs. Follow-up studies in 1947 showed that despite rationing and the psychological stresses of war, the health of Britain's domestic population had bloomed. A plain but balanced diet, Drummond had discovered, was the nearest thing to the elixir of life.

෪ ๖

THE WEEKLY RATION

Bacon and ham: 4 oz

Other meat: to the value of 1s 2d

Butter: 2 oz

Cheese: 2 oz

Margarine: 4 oz

Cooking fat: 4 oz

Milk: 3 pints + 1 packet dried skimmed milk per month

Sugar: 8 oz

Preserves: 1 lb every 2 months

Tea: 2 oz

Eggs: 1 shell egg + 1 packet dried egg per month

Sweets: 12 oz

෪ ๖

Drummond laid out his ground-breaking policy in an appendix to the Ministry of Food's import programme in May 1940, entitled *A Survey of War-time Nutrition*. As he knew from decades of research, Britain's pre-war diet had been adequate in what he called 'energy-rich foods' but short on 'protective' ones, especially those that supplied calcium, vitamins A and B1. The first course of action, therefore, was to step up home production of foodstuffs that provided those essentials, such as milk and vegetables. He also emphasized the importance of enough carbohydrates: he set the optimum calorie intake at 2500 for women and 3000 for men (slightly higher than the 2000–2500 range recommended for today's far more sedentary citizens).

His classification of food into simple types sounds an obvious course of action now, but in the 1940s it was revolutionary. The terms 'energy-rich' and 'protective' were still in standard use among food-writers many years later. Melissa's copy of *Mrs Beeton's Cookery and Household Management*, an updated edition from 1960 (but republished in 1979), made specific reference to them; it also spoke of the 'world events' that 'made vital an understanding of the principles of nutrition'. World War Two really was a turning point in the dietary education of the nation.

Drummond's wartime programme was accompanied by a brilliantly executed publicity campaign from the Ministry of Agriculture intended to persuade Britons to plant their own food. Under the patriotic banner slogan 'Dig for Victory', self-sufficiency became the new Holy Grail. Parks, gardens and grazing land were dug up or ploughed on an unprecedented scale. It was considered the duty of all householders to turn their back gardens into vegetable patches. Flowers were considered a frivolous use of earth, even in window boxes: proper patriots planted theirs with herbs and lettuce. Windsor Great Park was given over to wheat. Even Lord's cricket ground was not spared. Between 1939 and 1944, the arable land area in England and Wales increased by 63 per cent. Wheat, barley and potato crops almost doubled, while the production of oats rose by two-thirds. By the end of the war almost three-quarters of the food consumed in Britain was produced domestically, up from a third just six years before.

In a postscript to the BBC nine o'clock news at Christmas 1942, the Minister of Agriculture Robert Hudson was able to announce: 'Much hard work and technical skill have played their part in these mighty yields, amongst the richest of all time, but I believe we have a Higher Power to thank as well, and from the depths of our hearts. Some power has wrought a miracle in the English harvest fields this summer, for in this, our year of greatest need, the land has given us bread in greater abundance than we have ever known before.' God and the weather may have been kind to the farmers, but it was the Ministry of Food who had advised what needed to be grown. Drummond provided the science behind the spadework.

Because shipping space was at a premium, food imports also had to be drastically reorganized. Again at Drummond's instigation, priority was given to cheese, skimmed dried milk, tinned fish and meat, and pulses. He stopped the importation of fresh eggs in favour of a new dried variety. The import of nuts and fruit, with the exception of oranges, was reduced or (in the case of bananas) stopped altogether. Drummond argued that such foodstuffs took up too much space in relation to their nutritive value, or that there were easier ways of supplying the nutrients they contained, such as artificially fortifying margarine with specially imported concentrates of vitamins A and D. Meanwhile, with the German air-raids on Britain at their height, he devised a scientifically nourishing 'Blitz broth' that was served from mobile canteens to the survivors of the bombing and the auxiliary forces helping them. One cupful with a slice of bread was popularly held to be as good as a three-course meal. At one stage there were enough stocks of this broth held in secret storage around the country to feed 5 million people.

The technical ability to preserve food in cans had been mastered in the mid nineteenth century, but it was not until the 1940s that the process really took off. Canned food was airtight and therefore safe from contamination in the event of a poison gas attack by the Luftwaffe. Better still, from Drummond's point of view, was that canned food retained its vitamins. The contribution it could make to public nutrition in times of rationing was clear, and he promoted it tirelessly. Canned food eventually became so important that a Northern Irish chemist called A. J. Howard was appointed as Director of Canning at the Ministry. In 1949 Howard wrote a 287-page history of his subject called *Canning Technology*. With its obscure illustrations and chapter sub-headings such as 'Discolouration of the Interior of the Can and/or its Contents' and 'Determination of Thermal Death Times', *Canning Technology* was possibly one of the dullest books ever written, although Drummond, who provided the foreword, apparently did not find it dull at all. 'I do not know what proportion of those who write forewords actually read every word of the book they help to introduce,' he wrote, 'but I can assure Mr Howard [that] I was drawn by the magnetism of his clear and expert style to read it from beginning to end.'

With the contents of the nation's larder so radically rearranged, it was, of course, also necessary to alter the way people cooked – or in some instances to teach them to cook from scratch. The propaganda machine went into overdrive. Every morning the BBC broadcast 'Kitchen Front', a strange mixture of recipes, cooking tips and nutrition advice from a Radio Doctor. ('Health rule for April: It's a good idea to cook potatoes in their jackets. The skin stops the precious vitamin C from escaping and getting lost in the cooking water.') Ministry of Food-sponsored articles, advertisements, cartoons and slogans began to fill the newspapers, along with an unstoppable flood of official doggerel.

Some of this versification was cringe-making:

> I used to think one didn't oughter
> Make a soup from vegetable water.
> But this, my dear – this I S a snorter!

none of it was subtle:

> I saw three ships a-sailing
> But not with food for me.
> For I am eating home-grown foods
> To beat the enemy
> And ships are filled with guns instead
> To bring us Victory.

But the insistence on parsimony was remorseless:

> When salvage is all that remains of the joint
> And there isn't a tin and you haven't a "point"
> Instead of creating a dance and ballad
> Just raid the allotment and dig up a salad!

Even children were recruited to the cause:

> "Household" milk? Why, ma, that's easy:
> (Made this way, it can't go cheesy.)
> *First* the water, *then* the powder.'
> (Mother's never *quite* felt prouder!)

Humdrum vegetables underwent strange anthropomorphosis. Dr Carrot wore a top hat and half-moon glasses and carried a Gladstone bag with 'Vit A' written on it. Potato Pete, meanwhile, was a muscular farmer with a felt hat set at a jaunty angle and a barley stalk clamped in his teeth: '"I'll put pep in your step!" says Potato Pete.' The potato character was said to be very popular with children. Whether this was true or not, the scribes at the Ministry of Food again exerted themselves.

> *Song of Potato Pete*
> Potatoes new, potatoes old
> Potato (in a salad) cold
> Potatoes baked or mashed or fried
> Potatoes whole, potato pied
> Enjoy them all, including chips
> Remembering spuds don't come in ships!

The diet designed and promoted by Drummond was necessarily low-sugar, low-cholesterol, and often very inventive. The war generation still remembers such dishes as sausage and sultana casserole, carrot fudge, soyaghetti and, the most famous of all, Woolton Pie – a dish created by the head chef of the Savoy Hotel in May 1941 and that made up for its total absence of meat with plenty of swede and oatmeal.

இ் ்

WOOLTON PIE

Cooking time: about 1 hour

Quantity: 4 helpings

• This is an adaptable recipe that you can change according
to the ingredients you have available.

• Dice and cook about 1 lb each of the following in salted water:
potatoes (you could use parsnips if topping the pie with mashed
potatoes), cauliflower, swedes, carrots – you could add turnips too.
Strain but keep ¾ of a pint of the vegetable water.

• Arrange the vegetables in a large pie dish or casserole. Add a little
vegetable extract and about 1 oz rolled oats or oatmeal to the
vegetable liquid. Cook until thickened and pour over the vegetables;
add 3–4 chopped spring onions.

• Top with potato pastry or with mashed potatoes and a very little
grated cheese and heat in the centre of a moderately hot oven until
golden brown. Serve with brown gravy.

This is at its best with tender young vegetables.

LISTEN TO THE KITCHEN HOME FRONT AT 8.15 EVERY
MORNING

இ் ்

Drummond's achievement was essentially a complex juggling act. A
lesser man might easily have drowned in the political chicanery of an
emergency wartime government. His remit as the Ministry of Food's
Chief Scientific Adviser was far from clearly defined. He had to avoid
stepping on the toes of advisers in the Ministries of Agriculture and
Health. There was also established medical opinion to contend with,
because the conservative British Medical Association was frequently
wary of the MoF's new-fangled thinking.

Fortunately, Drummond was a talented committee man. He
promoted his arguments forcefully yet with a self-deprecating

friendliness so disarming that he almost always managed to get his way. His natural energy and enthusiasm had been a trademark since his time at university. Thomas Jeeves, Lord Horder, his co-adviser at the Ministry of Food (and a physician before and after the war to both George VI and Elizabeth II), wrote later that 'his tolerance, his humility and his insatiable desire for the truth never failed him, and he was for this reason the ideal colleague'.

Drummond saw opportunities for improvement everywhere, even in the nation's bread. In the type of white flour commonly used for bread before the war, many of the B vitamins present in the wheat berry were lost in the milling process. Drummond pushed hard for the introduction of wholemeal bread. His lobbying was so successful that by 1942, despite the protests of the Flour Millers' Association, white bread was removed altogether from the shelves and replaced with a variety known as the 'National Wheatmeal Loaf'.

> The Queen of Hearts
> Said 'No' to tarts
> There's Wheatmeal Bread for Tea.
> Each cream-gold slice
> Is oh, so nice
> And better far for me.

He paid special attention to society's 'vulnerable groups', as they were designated for the first time. Children and expectant or nursing mothers headed the list. In an echo of the experiments of William Stark, these groups received rations of blackcurrant and rosehip syrup as an alternative source of vitamin C, before concentrated orange juice became available – another first for Britain. Mothers and children also received rations of cod liver oil, and priority access to supplies of liquid milk when this, too, was rationed. The welfare of mothers and babies was doubtless a subject close to Drummond's heart: in 1942, two years after marrying

Anne Wilbraham, their daughter Elizabeth was born. He had become a father for the first time at the age of fifty-one.

Putting into practice what he had known in theory for more than twenty years must have been professionally satisfying for Drummond. As far back as 1918 he had published a paper on breast-feeding in which he noted the dangers of vitamin A deficiency in the nursing mother. He had discovered that what little vitamin A was present in the tissues of the breast was made available to the infant at the mother's expense, which made her very prone to infection, particularly of the eyes. His recommended remedy was a supplement of cod liver oil.

Adolescents were also generously treated. Proper meals were served in schools on a national basis for the first time. These had become necessary partly because so many mothers had left their homes to work in factories or as land girls. Extra rations were sent to schools along with cocoa and 'national milk'. The state's ⅓ pint milk allocation for school children, eventually enshrined in the School Milk Act of 1946, was to last for a quarter of a century. Its withdrawal in 1971 was deeply unpopular with the public, who gave the cost-cutting Education Secretary responsible the now famous nickname 'Maggie Thatcher, Milk Snatcher'. (I am just old enough to remember school milk and the tiny silver-top bottles it arrived in. The crates were delivered early and left on the school doorstep until break time, by when the milk was often unpleasantly tepid and turning to cream. We five-year-olds sometimes complained, but for the most part I secretly liked Drummond's school milk and was sorry when it disappeared from our daily routine.)

Some of Drummond's younger colleagues from the Ministry of Food are still alive today. The most famous of these by far is Marguerite Patten OBE, who joined the Ministry in 1942. Now in her nineties, she remains the leading authority on 1940s cuisine and the author of an extraordinary 170 cookery books, with worldwide sales of 17 million. She is also the country's oldest TV chef, having first cooked for the cameras in 1947, and she still makes regular appearances on television.

Not long before Jamie Oliver tackled the subject of school meals, I spotted Marguerite Patten in a documentary showing that modern British eight-year-olds typically consume 3000 calories a day: 1100 calories more than their counterparts ate in the 1940s (and, for eight-year-olds, 1100 calories more than is optimal). Needless to say, those 3000 calories tended not to come from healthy sources. Let loose in the school playground, the cameras panned over lunchboxes horrendously overfilled with confectionary, crisps and fizzy drinks.

Meanwhile in the school canteen, a control group of children were fed a wartime diet carefully recreated by Marguerite Patten over an eight-week period. She knew what she was doing: in 1942 the Ministry of Food had sent her to various school canteens to assess the food value and vitamin content of what was on offer. In the experiment sixty-two years later, tellingly enough, the crates of fresh vegetables delivered to the kitchen doors came from an expensive organic shop: the only way, Marguerite said, that the ingredients of wartime could faithfully be replicated. The children were suspicious of Marguerite's strange new offerings to start with, just as their counterparts had been in the 1940s, but the experiment's result was amazing. Some children grew one inch without putting on a single pound of weight. None of those following the modern diet lost weight or grew as dramatically, despite being the same age and attending the same London school.

∂∞ ∞

CORNED BEEF FRITTERS

Cooking time: 10 minutes	*Quantity*: 4 helpings
2 oz self-raising or plain flour	1 teaspoon grated onion
Pinch salt	1 teaspoon chopped parsley
1 egg yolk or ½ reconstituted egg	6 oz corned beef, finely flaked
½ gill milk or milk and water	1 oz clarified dripping or
Pinch dried mixed herbs	cooking fat

METHOD: Blend the flour with the salt, egg, and milk or milk and water. Beat until smooth batter then add the herbs, onion, parsley and corned beef. Melt the dripping or fat in a frying pan and when really hot drop in spoonfuls of the batter mixture. Fry quickly on either side until crisp and brown. Serve as soon as possible after cooking.

FOOD IS A MUNITION OF WAR. DON'T WASTE IT

ھ ⋞

I went to see Marguerite Patten at her brick-built bungalow in Withdean, a hilly suburb above Brighton. It was already a nostalgic part of the country for me. Withdean was near Devil's Dyke, a steep section of the South Downs where my parents used to take me on days out from boarding school, and where I once saw a hang-gliding enthusiast break his nose on take-off. Like the Dyke with its stupendous, Constable-celebrated view of the Sussex Weald, Withdean was quintessentially English. Its comfortable villas sported mock Tudor beams and fake leaded windows. One house even had a Union Jack flying above the porch. There were long views across the orderly terraces of Brighton proper to the glittering sea beyond.

It was the sort of place you would expect someone like Marguerite Patten to live. Literally as well as symbolically, this was the England that her generation had fought for. Spitfires once duelled with Messerschmitts in the skies where hang-gliders now silently wheeled. I had brought a trio of Marguerite's cookbooks to Withdean in the hope that she would sign them. One of them was called *We'll Eat Again*, and in her author photograph I fancied that she even looked a little like Vera Lynn.

She was unexpectedly petite in the flesh. Her bouffant coiffure, her pearls, the green velvet suit over a black-and-white silk blouse, her clipped accent – all of this was perfectly period. I had to ring several times before she answered the door because she was far deafer than she was prepared to admit. The lady was formidable despite her bird-like physique, and splendid in her pride.

'I'm afraid I can't give you much time,' she said, leading me briskly down the corridor. 'I'm expecting another journalist in half an hour.'

The walls in her immaculate sitting room were decorated with photographs, commemorative plates and a pair of water-colours all depicting Lancaster bombers. Marguerite's late husband, Bob, was a much-decorated gunnery officer who survived a remarkable eighty-four bombing missions in Lancasters. Barnes Wallis's Dambusters had been his friends. The water-colours on the wall were signed by 'Bomber' Harris himself.

Marguerite had been a 'home economist' in the electrical industry when the war started, a job that involved showing customers the full potential of new-fangled electric cookers. She joined the Ministry of Food's Advice Division in 1942, by then a network of 'food advice bureaus' had been established across the country. Thousands of shops were either bought or requisitioned and converted into demonstration theatres complete with a stage, chairs and mirrors for the audience. The bureaus usually included 'baby clinics' where real orange juice and extra powdered milk rations were distributed to new mothers.

'It was called national dried milk,' Marguerite said, 'and it came in a funny little mauve tin.'

The cleverness of the demonstration theatre was that it allowed Food Advice officers to interact with the public without dictating to them. The good ones, like Marguerite, loved the job because it let them impart their own enthusiasm for cooking. To begin with she was based in Cambridge: she recalled setting up her first demonstration stall in the town's market square, where she had to compete with the shouts of the regular fruit and vegetable sellers.

'The trick,' she said, 'was always to *tempt* people into eating new food. There was no point in trying to force them.'

Everyone knew that this approach, developed at MoF headquarters and rolled out across the nation through a series of training programmes, was the brainchild of Jack Drummond. As an experienced university teacher he knew that there was nothing to be achieved by talking down to the public.

'An ability to make nutrition easy to understand – that was his genius,' Marguerite said. 'This five-a-day fruit-and-veg regime that the authorities are pushing now won't work because it is too dictatorial. The government hasn't gone into it sensibly. People hate to be nannied.'

In late 1943 Marguerite graduated from Cambridge to London, where she took over the advice bureau at Harrods, performing two demonstrations every day. Soon afterwards she became a regular contributor on Kitchen Front radio, which proved to be the start of her extraordinarily long career in media cookery. I congratulated her on the recent school meals documentary I had seen her in. She replied that it was baffling to find herself back in fashion after so many years.

'Everyone is looking back these days. When I think of all the documentation, ration cards and so on, that I threw out after the war . . . I remember asking Bob about it at the time, and he said, "No, no-one will want any of that rubbish".'

The other journalist Marguerite had mentioned never turned up. I was pleased when the half-hour I had been promised extended to an hour, and then to an hour and a half. The old lady was mesmerizing to listen to; she relaxed and softened as she recalled the glory days of her 1940s youth.

'You should have seen the ladies at Harrods,' she laughed at one point, gripping my wrist with a tiny, claw-like hand. 'The smart ones sometimes put their noses in the air and walked straight past my cooking demonstrations – click, click, click in their shiny new heels. But they always sneaked in at the back of the audience for a little look later on. Oh yes!'

She asked me to wait a moment as I was saying goodbye, out on the damp and moss-encrusted porch, and reappeared with the phone number of someone she thought might have known Drummond personally at the Ministry of Food – a friend of hers called Louise Davies. I went around the corner and rang the number directly from my car.

'Jack Drummond?' said Louise Davies. 'Of course I remember him. A highly entertaining man, with a genuine passion for food. I had much admiration for his work on rationing. We all did. Things would have been very different without him. His murder was a terrible tragedy.'

She was a doctor who, like Marguerite, had made a long career out of dietary education. At the age of eighty-two she was still affiliated to the University of London's Gerontology Nutrition Unit. At twenty-one, and fresh from college, she was taken on at Ministry headquarters, a requisitioned mansion block in Portman Square just north of Oxford Street. Here she was put to work on a public information food magazine pitched at schools. The project, another of Drummond's ideas, was sophisticated for its time: its real intention, she explained, was to 'get to the parents' through the pupils, whom it was hoped would take the lessons of good nutrition home with them. Drummond, she said, was not always the easiest of bosses.

'He was a stickler for detail and he had a tendency to micro-manage the magazine. It was a relief when he passed control of it to Magnus Pyke. He was much more hands-off as an editor.'

It was clear that her years at the Ministry of Food had been as formative an experience as they had been for Marguerite Patten. The Ministry, she said, had been such a fun, zippy place to work. Magnus Pyke was known as an eccentric even then: when the public's donation of blood outstripped officialdom's ability to store it, he was rumoured to have suggested using the excess to make black pudding. The entire bureaucracy was shot through with a strong streak of Blitz Spirit – a cheery, roll-your-sleeves-up amateurism that Drummond both promoted and personified.

'It wasn't anything like a peacetime ministry. The hierarchy was very flexible because of the war, and it was full of poets and writers and other interesting people from outside the civil service.'

These included the novelist Lettice Cooper, aunt of Jilly Cooper's husband, who helped prepare scripts for the Kitchen Front broadcast, and Eileen O'Shaughnessy, the wife of George Orwell. (In his biography of Orwell, Bernard Crick remarked that the fictional Ministry of Truth in *Nineteen Eighty-Four* owed as much to O'Shaughnessy's experiences in the Ministry of Food as to Orwell's at the BBC.)

I later spoke to a third former Ministry employee called Joan Peters. From 1942 until the end of the war her workplace was a flat on the fourth floor of the Portman Square mansion block that had been converted into the Ministry's experimental kitchen – the laboratory, effectively, of the entire Woolton project. New recipes were tested here before being disseminated across the country. Drummond was naturally a frequent visitor to such an important cog in the machine.

'There were three of us girls in there: Mary, Sue and me, as well as Elvira McLeod, our boss,' Joan explained. 'Drummond was a handsome, friendly man. A gentleman, if you know what I mean . . . He was always very smart. With a moustache, rather like Anthony Eden.'

What she remembered most about him was his infectious enthusiasm.

'He was often in the kitchen asking Elvira's advice about something or other, or else in the press department down the corridor. He was always a great encouragement to us . . . the kitchen work was very hard, and there were endless air-raids and fire drills. It was a very wearying time.'

She experimented on several recipes such as eggless sponge, mock duck and parsley honey.

'You wouldn't believe how much parsley I had to chop,' she said. 'Oh my goodness me, what a lot of work.'

⤙ ⤚

PARSLEY HONEY

Cooking time: ¾ hour	*Quantity*: 1 lb
5 oz parsley (including stalks)	1 lb sugar
1½ pints water	½ teaspoon vinegar

METHOD: Pick parsley and wash well. Dry. Chop stalks up roughly. Put into a pan with 1½ pints of boiling water and boil until it reduces to a pint. Strain. Add 1 lb sugar and boil until syrupy (like honey) about 20 minutes, then add ½ teaspoonful of vinegar. Pour into pots and cover. This gels by the next day, and tastes and looks like heather honey.

THE MINISTRY OF FOOD WANTS YOUR COOKING SECRETS

ॐ ॐ

Recipes were not the only things subjected to experiment at Portman Square. Joan remembered helping to compile a recipe book for distribution by the Red Cross to POWs in Germany. It was full of useful tips such as how to make a cheese grater out of a tin can. Her kitchen was a showcase of British ingenuity. On one occasion she and the others were issued with clean overalls and told to expect a visit from a VIP. They stood to attention as a delegation headed by Eleanor Roosevelt swept in.

'She looked lovely. She had a black fox fur on with the head and tail clasped together, and a matching black hat . . . I think she liked our little kitchen very much indeed.'

It was easy to underestimate the achievement of public educators like Drummond, and to forget that in 1940 the word 'vitamin' was just twenty years old. To the public of the 1940s and 1950s, vitamins were almost magical. Dame Barbara Cartland, the world-record-breaking author of 723 mainly romantic novels, caught the public mood – or tried to – with a slim volume called *Vitamins for Vitality*, published in 1956. It was essentially a variation of the old food advice bureau format. 'Vitamin A is the *glamour vitamin*,' she wrote. 'If you know of an elderly woman whose skin, eyes and poise are those of a woman ten or twenty years younger, you can be sure that she enjoys a diet very rich in vitamin A . . . [it is] the Fountain of Youth for which men and women have sought since humanity could use its imagination.'

Vitamins are still credited with semi-mythical powers. The vitamin supplement industry is controversial in Britain and has been subjected recently to interference from Brussels, where regulators have questioned the efficacy and even the safety of hundreds of over-the-counter products. Yet a third of British women and a quarter of men still regularly take them in an industry worth £330m per year. Even more significant is the role of vitamins in the modern food industry's most controversial growth area: the sector known as nutraceuticals, or techno-foods. Processed food staples such as margarine, cereals and orange juice are fortified with vitamins and other 'scientific' ingredients associated with good health, and marketed to a credulous public who happily pay over the odds for them. Pepsi Co., for example, who own the juice brand Tropicana, sell an orange juice product called 'Multivitamins'; it costs five times more than ordinary orange juice. Unilever's Flora pro-activ margarine, meanwhile, contains hydrogenated sterols, a plant compound that is supposed to lower cholesterol in the blood; it costs eleven times as much as regular margarine. Nestlé, Danone and Kraft have all also invested heavily in the neutraceuticals sector, which was worth nearly $10bn worldwide in 2003 and was predicted to grow by 16 per cent a year.

Those figures would have surprised Drummond. He always argued that the best source of vitamins was natural food, and that so long as an individual's diet was plentiful and well balanced, supplements or additives were unnecessary. During the war, trials were conducted to determine whether supplementing the ration with vitamin pills improved health and physical well-being. 'No such effect was observed,' he commented in a lecture given to the Royal Institute of Chemistry in 1947. 'For the most part, prolonged vitamin therapy in the absence of obvious disease is useless.' (Half a century on, Kath Dalmeny of the consumer watchdog the Food Commission had this to say about the neutraceuticals sector: 'What the food industry is doing is taking out the wonderful nutrients nature provides in the right combinations, and sticking some of them into expensive products and pills and selling them back to us. You shouldn't need all this stuff if you are eating lots of fresh, plant-based foods.')

Like the ladies of the MoF who worked for him, Drummond believed that knowing how to cook was an essential of life, not a luxury. Thanks largely to his efforts, by 1945 an entire generation of housewives knew the rudiments of how to prepare a meal at home. They also knew a lot about vitamins – what they were, why they were important, and which foods contained them. The tragedy is how much of that hard-won knowledge has been forgotten. It was both absurd and tragic that Tony Blair's government was trying to educate the public all over again with its proposed 'traffic-light' labels on food packaging, a scheme intended to warn consumers about high levels of salt, sugar and fat. The initiative was controversial. Some critics thought the approach was too simplistic, others that it was another egregious example of New Labour's nanny state tendencies at work. The big supermarket chains naturally hated it and were threatening a boycott. But it seemed to me that the traffic-light system wouldn't have been necessary at all if the British public had remembered all or even some of what their grandparents had learned about food.

In 1935, Drummond wrote the preface to a book called *The Schoolboy – His Nutrition and Development*, which showed that the incidence of bone fractures among boys at Christ's Hospital school rose when margarine replaced butter in 1917, and fell again when butter was restored in 1922. 'It is a fact at once surprising and humiliating,' he wrote, 'that with thousands of years of human life and experience behind us we are actually engaged today in acquiring laboriously the knowledge necessary to enable us to feed and rear our children properly.' Using a rather different vocabulary, Jamie Oliver was saying precisely the same thing seventy years later. Thanks in part to Drummond, bone fractures among schoolchildren are no longer a problem. And yet, as Jamie Oliver pointed out in his TV series, we have still not learned how to feed our children properly.

The MoF ladies do not blame today's parents for their culinary ignorance. Their opprobrium was reserved mainly for the successive Departments of Education who had consistently refused to acknowledge the importance of learning how to cook. They felt that the discipline had been squeezed into an ever-tighter corner over the last quarter century, robbed of all glamour and denuded of funding. 'Domestic Science', as cookery was once called, was never more than an optional extra on the school curriculum. Domestic Science was rebranded 'Home Economics' in the early 1970s in a bid to make the subject sound more modern and egalitarian. For twenty years it was possible to take a Home Economics O-Level in Cookery and Nutrition. Melissa, for one, had taken the exam in 1985 (and was naturally awarded an A), but in 1990 a reform-minded Conservative government sought to cut cookery from the curriculum altogether.

'They justified the decision by saying that mothers don't cook these days because they are too busy working,' Joan Peters said, 'but that's a crazy argument. If the parents don't know what's good for their children, how are the children supposed to learn?'

Cookery in any form would have disappeared from the curriculum altogether if it weren't for NATHE, the National Association for Teachers of Home Economics. Their lobbyists 'saved' it by bringing the topic under the curricular umbrella of Design and Technology, which had been declared a compulsory subject. These days, the nearest a state-educated child can usually get to learning how to cook is to take an option called 'Food Technology' – a course that focuses on packaging and processing rather than on skills in the kitchen, and that lays heavy emphasis on 'industrial practice'. As a consequence, nutrition has become a subset of a subset of a minor academic field, while learning how to cook per se isn't taught at all.

꙳ ꙳

DESIGN AND TECHNOLOGY
(FOOD TECHNOLOGY)
PAPER NUMBER 4

Additional materials: None

Candidates answer on the question paper

Time 1 hour 15 minutes

1. In a factory making frozen lasagne, particular care has to be taken
in separating raw materials from the finished product.

a) Give three reasons why this is necessary.

b) A HACCP (Hazard Analysis and Critical Control Point) system is
set up to ensure product safety. List three HACCP checks that would
be carried out during the production of the frozen lasagne.

c) Computer control is used by the manufacturer to ensure quality
of the frozen lasagne. List four ways that computer systems can
assist the manufacturer in this process.

(From the first page of a GCSE exam paper, 2003)

꙳ ꙳

Drummond was lionized for his role in turning the nation's
housewives into an army of real cooks. His knighthood in 1944 was
greeted with broad popular acclaim. 'He is a back-room boy of a different
type,' ran one gushing newspaper article of 1946, beneath the headline
'The Only Sir Jack'. 'He refuses to be called Sir John, and thinks up special
hates for friends who call him Cecil, his second name . . . While others
were thinking up bigger and better bombs, he was shut away in his
laboratory thinking up smaller and more nutritious meals.'

In reality, Drummond was seldom to be found shut away in his or
anybody else's laboratory. It simply wasn't his style. Besides, his role at
the Ministry of Food changed and expanded as the pressure on shipping
in the Atlantic diminished and the war entered its final phase. By the time
of Eleanor Roosevelt's visit to Portman Square, his reputation had been

established internationally. The food supplies that at last began to flow from America under the Lend-Lease Act could not easily be administered from a desk in London. Drummond was obliged to visit the US on several occasions, and so was the natural candidate to represent British interests at the Hot Springs Conference in Virginia in June 1943 – a conference that led to the formation of UNFAO, the United Nations Food and Agriculture Organization. For the first time in history, the business of feeding people was about to be tackled on a global level.

The US was not his only foreign destination during the war. In early 1942 he was asked to send someone to besieged Malta to look into the worsening food situation there. Drummond evidently didn't want for courage, and went himself rather than put someone else in danger. He was able to make several important practical suggestions, including the immediate airlifting of a ton of ascorbic acid and the recommendation that children be fed vitaminized chocolate, before being flown off the island in a lull between air-raids. Lord Gort, the Commander-in-Chief on Malta, declared that it was thanks to Drummond that starvation never took significant hold during the siege.

Drummond was evidently not the sort to confine himself to dispensing advice and theory from the safety of the rear. From D-Day onwards, his attention turned increasingly to the continent and its starving millions who had not had the benefit of his scientifically organized diet. In May 1945 he travelled in secret with a party of other scientists and doctors through the collapsing enemy lines in the western Netherlands. He found a population subsisting on sugar beet and fried tulip bulbs, and teetering on the brink of mass starvation. Some 30,000 people had already starved to death during the notorious 'Hongerwinter' of 1944. Negotiation with the German occupiers led to Operation Manna, in which RAF Lancasters swapped their bouncing bombs for K-rations and air-dropped some 7000 tons of food to the starving Dutch in a single week. Drummond was on hand to advise which food should be sent where. Among those saved was the sixteen-year-old Audrey Hepburn –

Edda Van Heemstra, as she called herself then – who was languishing in the ruins of Arnhem with her Dutch mother. Without Drummond there would perhaps have been no *Breakfast at Tiffany's*.

The experience of Operation Manna led him to develop an easily digested porridge for the emergency treatment of the seriously starved. Known as 'Drummond mixture', it was deployed at Bergen-Belsen and other Nazi death camps as they were liberated, and undoubtedly saved thousands of lives. In January 1945 he published a manual called *Nutrition and Relief Work*, which became the standard text for the armies of the Liberation. Drummond saw the horrors of Bergen-Belsen for himself, a month after its inmates had been freed. The Dutch later made him a Commander of the Order of Orange Nassau. The Netherlands was not the only country to acknowledge his contribution to civilian welfare. The University of Paris conferred on him the degree of Doctor *honoris causa*; Washington awarded him the US Medal of Freedom (with Silver Palms); New York elected him an Honorary Member of the Academy of Sciences.

The working-class orphan from Charlton had come further than he or anyone else could possibly have anticipated. When the war ended the 54-year-old found himself in a position of extraordinary power and influence. An internationally recognized authority on nutrition, he was a knight of the realm who counted lords and government ministers among his friends. As a Fellow of the Royal Society he was an acknowledged pillar of the scientific establishment. Modest, likeable and a proven war hero, he had the kind of profile that modern politicians can only dream about. Even his name sounded heroic: his fictional namesake, Bulldog Drummond, was the 1920s creation of Herman Cyril McNeile, whose hugely popular novels were subtitled 'The Adventures of a Demobilized Officer Who Found Peace Dull'.

The real Drummond cannot have found the prospect of peace dull. On the contrary, it represented an opportunity enjoyed by no other biochemist in history. Ever since he was a young man his ambition had been to improve standards of public nutrition. By 1945 he had achieved that goal and seemed to be in an ideal position to make permanent the extraordinary changes he had brought about. That should have been his legacy. Instead, Britain has all but forgotten how to cook and to eat, and Drummond is usually remembered – when he is remembered at all – as the victim in a squalid tabloid murder story. His awful death eclipsed as well as truncated an apparently exemplary life. His entry in the *Chambers Biographical Dictionary* ran to just one line – 'DRUMMOND, Sir Jack Cecil: See DOMINICI, Gaston', it said – while DOMINICI, Gaston was granted a whole paragraph. Where did it all go so wrong? If ever a reputation was ripe for rehabilitation, it seemed to me that Jack Drummond's was it.

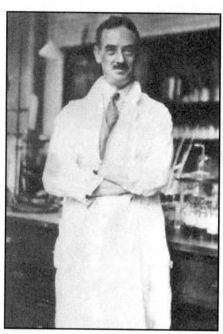

*Jack Drummond in his laboratory at
UCL, early 1930s*

Chapter 2

The Way We Eat Now

'If Foods contribute so necessarily to the Preservation of Life and Health, they also produce the greatest Part of those Distempers, to which we are subject, and many Times, by the ill Use of them, cause even Death itself. All which being set together, we may easily see, that the Ground-work of our Preservation, consists chiefly in a knowledge of suiting Foods to every Constitution, as it best agrees with it; and so the Knowledge we ought to be most desirous of, should be that of Foods.'

Louis Lemery, *A Treatise of all Sorts of Foods* (1745),

quoted in *The Englishman's Food*

Until I met Melissa I treated the business of eating a bit like filling up a car with petrol. The body was a machine to be refuelled; eating was a chore to be completed as quickly and as cheaply as possible. It wasn't that I didn't like good food. It was more that I didn't necessarily dislike bad food, either. I was an undiscerning consumer who didn't question the quality of what I was putting in my mouth any more than the consistency of the petrol that came out of the forecourt pumps. Tesco was the same to me as Texaco; I didn't much differentiate between a pure pork chipolata from Smithfield's Market and an ersatz product from Iceland. But my attitude began to change when Melissa playfully held up a mirror to my blithe bachelor ways. She weaned me off the processed ready-meals on which I had been subsisting for years mainly by making me read the labels on the packaging, and before long I was as curious about what was in my food as she had trained herself to be. We were in love; and in 2004 we married and went on honeymoon to America.

'This place,' said Melissa, 'is a disgrace.'

We were standing on the Strip in Las Vegas beneath a large billboard advertising vasectomy reversal ('Call 1-713-R E V E R S E – Money Back Guarantee'). But it wasn't that, or the unfettered gambling, or any other of Sin City's shameless excesses that had prompted her outburst: it was the fatties. Drummond would have been stunned by the crisis of obesity across the Atlantic. When it came to bad eating habits, the chips-through-the-railings episode filmed by Jamie Oliver was as nothing compared to what was going on in the western United States.

Melissa and I were familiar in theory with America's waistline statistics, but seeing what these meant in practice still came as a shock. It was like visiting the Grand Canyon for the first time: nothing had quite prepared us for the extraordinary scale of it. The rate of obesity among adults in the American heartlands was running at 30 per cent – about double what it had been on my last visit to this part of the country in the 1980s. The proof was everywhere: in the casinos of Las Vegas, in the car parks at beauty spots, in the restaurants across the four states we visited – most of all in the restaurants. We invented a private game called 'Who ate all the pies?', which involved much smirking and rolling of the eyes. Yet, after a while, the game didn't seem so funny. The fattest of the fatties were not amusing but grotesque. It was certain that some of these unfortunates weren't going to live for very long: the strain on their hearts was simply too great.

The reasons weren't hard to spot. Most obviously, the size of the portions served in the restaurants bore no resemblance to anything found in western Europe. There was often too much even for the greediest customers, who routinely asked for a doggie bag to take home what they could not manage. The waiters were unflustered: the bags were always on hand. Doggie bags had become a normal part of the

American dining experience. Melissa and I quickly learned to order for one and then share.

The other obvious reason was the dearth of decent food. We drove 3000 miles in the course of our road trip-cum-honeymoon and discovered vast tracts of land where there really was nothing to eat but junk. On one memorable day we went out of our way to find fresh fruit and vegetables, but ended up in a fast-food outlet consuming strawberry milkshakes and deep-fried onion rings.

One hot afternoon on the outskirts of Albuquerque, New Mexico, we stopped at a gas station to buy drinking water. The attached convenience store looked shabby, but inside we found three long rows of state-of-the-art refrigerators containing nothing but fizzy drinks. Our European eyes were dazzled by the choice on display. We counted at least fifty brands for sale, and their very names seemed marvellous to us. Where else but in America could you find drinks called *Barg's*, *Blue Sky* and *Baja Bob's*, *Mello Yello* and *Mr Pibb*, *Squirt* and *Surge* and *Think!*? (Later, in Mormon Utah, we fell about laughing over a brand of beer called *Polygamy Porter*: 'Why just have one?' said the label.) Like Augustus Gloop, the boy-glutton in Roald Dahl's *Charlie and the Chocolate Factory*, I rather wanted to try them all. Melissa was made of sterner stuff, though: she just wanted a bottle of water. She shuttled up and down scanning every frosted window, but eventually gave up and had to ask at the counter.

'Water?' said the check-out woman. 'We don't sell water here. This is a convenience store. Maybe you could ask a mechanic.'

'It's not for the car, it's for me.'

'Oh, you mean *drinking* water! Well, pardon me . . . I guess maybe we don't sell it, but you're welcome to use the bathroom. Where are you guys from anyway?'

The nearest they had to H_2O was an isotonic activity drink called *Sport Water*. Melissa bought a bottle anyway, mainly out of politeness, but secretly pulled a face at me as she tasted it. It was heavily flavoured with fruit and very sweet. Then we looked more closely at the drinks in the refrigerators and discovered that virtually every one contained a sweetener of some kind. The most popular by far was an additive seldom seen in Europe called HFCS: High Fructose Corn Syrup. We had already discovered that we didn't much like drinks flavoured with HFCS, a substance six times sweeter than cane sugar. To our palates they were just too sweet. Furthermore, they all seemed to taste the same. In the convenience store we saw for the first time that the choice on offer was illusory. Even the *Sport Water* was really just another fizzy drink without the colour. We felt like the victims of a clever marketing trick in which the only thing that varied was the packaging, never the product.

We had both read Eric Schlosser's *Fast Food Nation*, so had some understanding of how all this had come about. Now, at a bookstore in Santa Fe, we bought Greg Critser's *Fatland* and began to find out more, taking turns to read out the choicest bits while the other drove. The reason American drinks manufacturers used HFCS in their products was because corn was cheap. 'In what would prove to be one of the single most important changes to the nation's food supply,' wrote Greg Critser, '[in 1984] both Coke and Pepsi switched from a fifty-fifty blend of sugar and corn syrup to 100 per cent HFCS. The move saved both companies 20 per cent in sweetener costs, allowing them to boost portion sizes and still make substantial profits.'

Never mind that HFCS was blamed by many scientists for contributing directly to America's obesity epidemic. (Research has shown that the human liver is unable to break fructose down in the normal way, and instead converts it straight into fat.) Never mind either that it was an inferior-tasting sweetener that cloyed unpleasantly on the tongue: American soda-pop drinkers had known little else for over twenty years and had acquired quite a taste for it. Research showed that the average American consumed the equivalent of fifty-three teaspoons of sugar a day. There was even some evidence that HFCS was addictive. But in America, it seemed, portion size and profit margins mattered more than public health, and quantity was often substituted for quality, even at the top end of the restaurant business.

Near the end of our honeymoon we stopped in Flagstaff, Arizona, and went out to dinner at a restaurant recommended by all the guidebooks as the best for many miles around. We were overjoyed by the deliciousness of the steaks, and reassured by the expensiveness of the wine list, but when Melissa asked for some cheese to accompany the last bit of a bottle of Californian Merlot, the waiter looked puzzled.

'Cheese?'

'Yes please,' she said. 'Whatever you've got.'

'I'll speak to the chef,' he replied.

There was a long wait. When he reappeared he was proudly bearing a tray of small yellow cubes, each of which had been speared with a cocktail stick. It was Monterrey Jack, the bland and rubbery substance used everywhere in America for melting across hamburgers. This was as good an illustration as any of the gulf of understanding between Europe and the US when it came to fine dining, although what astonished us at the time was the enormous size of the tray. As Melissa remarked, there were enough cheese cubes arranged on it to feed a small drinks party. It looked like a fakir's bed of nails.

From the dietary point of view it was a relief to return to London. With the memory of America fresh in mind, however, Melissa and I couldn't help but notice that the newspapers were filled with dire warnings that obesity was on the rise in Europe, too.

'It seems the Yanks didn't eat all the pies after all,' Melissa said one day. 'Just look at this.'

We were staying at her stepfather's house in Twickenham. It was breakfast time – a meal I had never much bothered with before I met Melissa – and she was reading her mother's copy of the *Daily Mail* at the kitchen table while I ate a new-regime kipper.

'It says here that obesity levels in Britain are rising faster than anywhere else in the world. Can that really be true?'

I glanced over her shoulder at the newspaper's headline: 'JUNK FOOD TIMEBOMB', it read.

'Typical *Mail* scare-story,' I replied. 'You can't believe half of what that paper says.'

'It's not the *Mail* who's saying it. It's the Royal College of Physicians. Apparently, unless something is done soon to reverse the trend, the life expectancy of the next generation could be lower than their parents.'

'The end of civilization as we know it, then.'

'Oh, just eat your kipper.'

I read the article for myself later and found that, just for once, the *Mail*'s apocalyptic tone was possibly justified. There was no arguing with the statistics that its report drew on. The television programme-makers' recent focus on school meals was no gimmick: obesity was a bigger problem in the UK than I had ever suspected. Britain's cultural emulation of America was almost axiomatic for my generation, but it was still surprising to learn that we were copying their obesity problems too. Junk food was sold on every British high street, but unlike some of the places we had just visited on honeymoon there was no obligation to live on it. Nevertheless, adult obesity in Britain had trebled in the last twenty-five years, to 22 per cent of the population. This meant that heart disease, a comparative rarity fifty years ago, was now our number-one killer, while the incidence of Type 2 diabetes, another condition closely linked to obesity, had risen by 450 per cent since 1960. What was happening to the nation's children was even more insidious: one in twelve six-year-olds and one in seven fifteen-year-olds were now obese. The Royal College of Physicians reckoned that more than half the country could be obese by the 2020s, a forecast that one nutritionist was calling 'an epidemic of proportions not seen since the plague'.

Increased life expectancy was an important yardstick of Western development. The *Mail* was talking about a demographic change without modern precedent: it seemed scarcely credible that civilization was on the point of going backwards. I wondered what Drummond would have made of the crisis. Our car-centred, exercise-free lifestyle was obviously part of the trouble, but the *Mail* was surely right to identify cheap junk food as the greater source of the problem. As a nation, we urgently needed to recapture the knowledge of how to eat properly if Britain was to avoid succumbing to a plague-like epidemic of fat. Here was another good reason to continue pursuing the Drummond story. The nutritive values he once promoted could hardly be more relevant. The monster of 'dietetic ignorance' that he had sought to slay in the 1940s was now literally killing us. I ordered a copy of the Royal College of Physicians' report, which was called *Storing up Problems – The Medical Case for a Slimmer Nation*; but not long afterwards, in the summer of 2004, life intervened to distract me from my new project.

Melissa was pregnant. The excitement we felt at the prospect of first-time parenthood was accompanied by a frenzied reorganization of our lives. She sold her one-bedroom flat, I rented out mine, and with our resources pooled we found a bigger place and busied ourselves in our new nest.

Meanwhile, my own dietary education changed up a gear. The cooking and eating of food both at home and in restaurants had been an important part of our relationship from its outset – food was Melissa's job, after all – but when she became pregnant the question of diet moved forcefully into the centre of our lives. The pregnancy manuals that rapidly piled up on her bedside table were filled with admonitions to eat well. I had not previously appreciated the power and influence of this literary genre. The zeal with which she set about turning dietary theory into practice was amazing. She seemed to have embarked on an almost sacred mission to purify her body. The days when she drank cider by the pint and smoked Marlboro reds were decisively over. She dutifully avoided alcohol and shellfish, ate five portions of fruit and vegetables a day as the government recommended, and swallowed the approved dose of folic acid supplement – although she questioned the need for that.

'If folic acid is so important for healthy foetal development, how come I can't get it from my ordinary food?' she wanted to know. 'It's only vitamin B9. You can get that from all sorts of vegetables – asparagus, broccoli, spinach. I don't understand why the government is so keen on artificial supplements.'

It was a good point. The British nation had reached the twenty-first century without dying out. It made one wonder where all the natural folic acid had got to. The government's recommendation seemed tantamount to an admission that the national diet was deficient.

One day, while shopping together at the supermarket, we reached a kind of impasse. I'd put a bottle of concentrated lemon juice in the trolley. Melissa took one look at the label and put it back on the shelf.

'What's wrong with that? It's only lemon juice.'

'If you want lemon juice, buy a lemon,' she said.

'But I don't want a lemon. I only want the juice!'

'It's got preservatives in it. I don't want "2-methyl-3-(pisopropylphenyl)-propionaldehyde" in my body, thanks very much.'

'But vitamin C is good for you.'

'We've got to cut down on preservatives.'

'We'll probably get scurvy,' I grumbled.

But Melissa had thought of that. Back at home she placed a weekly fruit and veg order with an organic delivery company. She also announced that, henceforth, we would be shopping for meat and fish in the local farmer's market.

'I think you're in danger of becoming an orthorexic.'

'You and your orthorexia,' she said, rolling her eyes. 'All I can say is I'd rather be an orthorexic than give birth to a baby with three legs and a fatal allergy to peanuts.'

Orthorexia nervosa was a new eating disorder that I had just discovered on the Internet, and it was my contention that it deserved much wider public recognition. The condition was identified in 1997 by Stephen Bratman, a nutritionist from Colorado. Orthorexics, he claimed, were characterized by a 'grim sense of self-righteousness' and a mindset that 'begins to consume all other sources of joy and meaning'; they 'reach a point where they spend most of their lives planning, purchasing, preparing and eating meals'. Severe sufferers developed such a fixation on food quality that they ended up rejecting everything, and in a few extreme cases had starved themselves to death. I didn't really think Melissa or I were in danger of that, but the early symptoms of the condition were still recognizable in her product label-reading. I was convinced that orthorexia, or at least a mild form of it, was a common affliction among modern supermarket shoppers. The term had yet to enter the lexical mainstream, but I was sure it wouldn't be long. *Bulimia nervosa* was not recognized as a clinical condition until 1979, after all.

Orthorexia struck me as symptomatic of a deepening crisis in the West's relationship with its food. The most obvious indicator was that tabloid newspaper staple, the food scare. Until the late 1980s these were a relative novelty in Britain. Food scares were something that happened to hysterical foreigners, not the phlegmatic British. In the US in 1959, for example, it was revealed that Aminotriazole, a weed-killer widely used on cranberries, produced cancer of the thyroid in rats. Although it was reported that a human would need to eat thousands of pounds of cranberries to produce the same result, the then Secretary of State for Health, Arthur S. Fleming, advised that housewives should avoid buying cranberries as a precaution, pending further tests. His comment, two weeks before Thanksgiving and its traditional dinner of turkey and cranberry sauce, could not have been more ill-timed, and ultimately cost Congress $10m in compensation payments to fruit-growers.

In 1988, however, it became Britain's turn when Edwina Currie, a junior health minister under Margaret Thatcher, commented that most of Britain's eggs were contaminated with salmonella. Some 400 million eggs had to be destroyed as demand collapsed. The scare also cost 4 million hens their lives, and Edwina Currie her job. Public confidence in Britain's food supply never quite recovered: by the 1990s, food scares had become commonplace. Salmonella in eggs was followed by 'listeria hysteria' in cheese. In 1995 the first human case of Creuzfeldt-Jakob Disease was reported, a fatal disease thought to be linked to Bovine Spongiform Encephalytis, or Mad Cow Disease. The livestock industry was decimated by a three-year ban on exports to the EU. In 1996, an outbreak of E-coli poisoning in meat products in Lanarkshire killed twenty-one people. A record 100,000 official cases of food poisoning were reported in Britain in the same year, although some scientists claimed the true figure was ten times higher.

Food scares had become part of the backdrop of modern life, and 2004 turned out to be a bumper year. We were deluged with media reports about everything from unauthorized chemicals in farmed Scottish salmon to the dye used in chicken tikka masala and prawn cocktail-flavoured crisps. Even water was no longer above suspicion when it emerged that Coca-Cola's new brand of water, Dasani – 'as pure as bottled water gets', according to its marketing men – was actually taken from the mains at their plant in Sidcup. What was worse, Coca-Cola's bottling process managed to introduce illegal levels of carcinogenic bromate into their over-packaged product.

In a rational world, public confidence in the bottled water market should have been severely shaken by the Dasani scandal. In the real world, sales were not just unaffected: they continued to boom. Britons spent £1.6bn on bottled water in 2004, up from £360m in 1998, and were expected to spend more than £2bn by 2010. Melissa and I drank a good deal of bottled water, and her reaction to the Dasani scandal was complex. First, she bought a new kettle with a built-in filter. The purchase was perfectly logical. According to consumer groups, the quality of mains water in south-east England was as high as anywhere in Europe. As Coca-Cola must have realized, it was indistinguishable from mineral water once it was filtered. It also came out of the taps at about one-thousandth of the cost. On the other hand, bottled water did not disappear from the weekly shopping list. Melissa continued to buy the fizzy kind, which she liked to drink with lime juice. This was fair enough. However, she also continued occasionally to buy bottles of the still variety, particularly Evian, in spite of our fancy new kettle.

'I *like* Evian,' she explained when I pointed out the contradiction. 'The bottles come cold from the fridge, and they're good to have by the bed at night.'

When I suggested putting a jug of filtered tap-water in the fridge and taking that to bed, she replied only that this 'wouldn't be the same'.

I was puzzled by the public's indifference to what was happening to our food supply generally. It was as though the media had cried 'wolf' so often that the public were no longer scared by food scares. In fact the worse the food scare, the more determinedly blinkered the public seemed to become. The Sudan 1 scandal was a case in point. In 2003, the Food Standards Agency was forced to recall hundreds of food products from supermarket shelves after they were found to contain Sudan 1, a red dye linked to cancer and prohibited across the EU. Manufactured in Asia, the dye was more usually found in solvents, petrol and shoe polish, but somehow found its way into a batch of chili powder used by Premier Foods to manufacture Worcester sauce. The sauce was then used as an ingredient in everything from Asda's *Good For You* BBQ chicken wedges and Morrison's *Eat Smart* cottage pie (frozen), to Sainsbury's *Be Good To Yourself* thousand island dressing and Tesco's *Healthy Living* sausage and mash. Two years later the FSA was still discovering food products containing the dye, and had ordered the withdrawal of some 580 different lines. It was the biggest product recall in British supermarket history. Yet, once again, confidence in processed foods did not collapse or even dip.

The media were perhaps complicit in the public's lack of concern. From the newspaperman's point of view, the Sudan 1 story was the *wrong kind* of food scare. Like the war in Bosnia, it was too drawn-out and too complicated for the public to understand easily. Perhaps, also, the implications of something so disastrous, so close to home, were too uncomfortable to deal with. For whatever reason, the story was soon relegated to the inside pages, just as the Bosnian war once was. Like the Dasani scandal, it barely blipped on the radar of national consciousness.

It undoubtedly blipped on ours. By now a year had passed since I had eaten a supermarket ready-meal, and a box of organic groceries was turning up on our doorstep every week. It was an increasingly fashionable way to shop in London, according to the consumer magazines, which automatically made me wary: my inclination was to resist faddishness on principle. Yet even I could see that the box's contents were as good as anything in the organic foods section at the supermarket, and I soon became an enthusiastic convert. The potatoes were always muddy, the fruit was often blemished, and the broccoli contained the occasional caterpillar – I half-suspected that the delivery company put them in to prove that their goods were pesticide-free – but it all tasted fine once it was cleaned. Most of it, moreover, was local. It was also seasonal, unlike the organic broccoli that for some reason was available all the year round at Tesco. Melissa also reckoned that, fruit for fruit and vegetable for vegetable, home delivery was actually cheaper than buying organic in the supermarket.

'It's amazing, considering how the supermarkets bang on about what good value they are. How come everyone in London doesn't buy groceries like this?'

'I don't know,' said Melissa. 'Force of habit? The power of advertising? Or maybe people are frightened of caterpillars.'

'They ought to be more worried about chemicals. The way the risk of Sudan 1 has been downplayed is just plain weird.'

I was thinking of a government expert called Alan Boobis, whose comment that the risk of eating foods adulterated with Sudan 1 was 'equivalent to the risk associated with smoking one cigarette in a lifetime' had been widely reported in the press. It was a clever comparison, and as an eminent toxicologist at Imperial College, London, Boobis carried a certain authority. However, he was also a member of the parliamentary advisory committee on the carcinogenicity of chemicals in food, which made me wonder about the objectivity of his media-friendly remark.

As Health Secretary Fleming learned to his cost during the Great American Cranberry Scare of 1959, governments have a strong interest in dispelling public fears over chemical contamination of the food supply – a rather greater interest, possibly, than in dealing with the contaminants themselves. For example, there had been no pronouncement from the FSA on the subject of Acrylamide, a carcinogen produced when foods high in starch are cooked or processed at high temperatures, such as crisps; and yet Acrylamide is more carcinogenic than Sudan 1. As another expert, Dr Erik Millstone, remarked, 'There is a great contrast between the urgency with which the FSA are moving on Sudan 1, and Acrylamide where the evidence of toxicity is stronger. Instead of naming and shaming products with Acrylamide, the FSA is just working behind the scenes with industry to try to reduce them.'

In other words the FSA, a supposedly independent body set up by the government after the Mad Cow crisis specifically in order to protect the public's health and consumer interests in relation to food, was at best inconsistent in its pronouncements on food safety; at worst, it was guilty of deliberately keeping the public out of the information loop. No doubt they had their reasons, but the tactic still seemed an unnecessarily long way from the simple food advice disseminated by Jack Drummond in the 1940s. No wonder the public was confused – and no wonder so many people found it easier to let others take responsibility for the safety of what they ate, or simply to ignore the issue.

The most obvious way to avoid chemical contamination was to switch, as Melissa and I had, to eating organic food. Plenty of people in Britain had done the same: the country's organics market was rising faster than in any other country in Europe. Yet for all the hype, organic food still only accounted for 1.2 per cent of the total British retail food market. In 2005, Britons spent £1.6bn on organic produce: only fractionally more than what we spent on bottled water. Despite all the warnings and an explosion of food scares, the vast majority of people were simply carrying on as before.

The scare over farmed Scottish salmon offered further evidence of the public's curious apathy. I loved salmon and so did Melissa. Salmon in a teriyaki marinade – on a bed of wasabi mash – was one of her signature dishes. But now a group of American scientists led by Ronald Hites of Indiana University was claiming that Scotland's farmed variety was the most chemically contaminated in the world. Levels of fourteen banned chemical substances were found to be so high that eating it more than three times a year was said to increase the risk of cancer. Given that oily fish such as salmon has been considered since Drummond's time to be essential for human health, this was quite a claim. Even now, the FSA recommends that pregnant women should eat two portions of oily fish a week.

I followed the story carefully in the newspapers. The way it was reported copied a familiar pattern. One bunch of scientists claimed farmed salmon was dangerous; another bunch asserted that it wasn't. The farmers complained that the testing methods were unfair; the FSA insisted that the potential risks were 'minimal', and were in any case outweighed by the health benefits of eating oily fish. The headlines faded after the usual two or three weeks, leaving the argument unresolved and the public in the dark.

Not long afterwards I went with Melissa to Billingsgate in east London, the country's principal fish market, where she had a meeting with a supplier known as Chris the Fish, one of Billingsgate's biggest operators. I had gone along to keep her company, and to see if Melissa's claim that the market café's kippers were the best in London was true. It was five o'clock in the morning and still dark outside, but noise and light streamed from the giant sheds along West India Quay. Fork-lift trucks scooted, doors slammed, pallets crashed. Stall-holders whistled cheerfully or called out to their mates in fruity Cockney, stamping their white rubber boots in the puddles on the slick concrete floor. Porters weaved in and out, their breath turning to vapour in the chilly air, their backs bent against the weight of trolleys stacked with crated seafood.

Chris the Fish wanted to show us around. It seemed a good opportunity to learn something about the salmon scare at first hand.

'It's just a bunch of scientists arguing on paper,' Chris said. 'They don't know a thing. Of course salmon isn't poisonous.'

'Excuse my French but it's a load of fackin' bollocks,' an angry voice interrupted. This was Mick, a crab specialist. A jowly, rough-looking man in dirty dungarees and a roll-neck sweater, he came out from behind a gently collapsing hillock of crustaceans and slapped a fat hand on my shoulder.

'I'll tell you straight,' he growled. 'You'd have to eat your body weight in salmon every week before the chemicals would harm you. *Every week.* That's a scientific fact.'

It didn't sound very scientific to me. The argument was uncannily similar to that used by the defenders of the pesticide used on cranberries in the 1950s, and of the red food-dye Sudan 1.

'I wonder if anyone has ever actually tried to eat their body weight in salmon,' I began. 'It would be an interesting experiment. Have you ever heard of William Stark? He was this Glaswegian bloke in the seventeenth century who ate nothing but honey puddings . . .'

Melissa silenced me with a jab in the ribs.

'No-one's ever died of eating fish from Billingsgate, see?' Mick continued, 'No-one. And in my opinion these so-called experts should shut up. It's messing with people's livelihoods!'

We moved on through the market.

'Sorry about that,' said Chris when we were out of earshot. 'Mick gets a bit emotional but he's basically right. This salmon scare is a load of bollocks. The public understands: they just ignore it. Salmon sales haven't been affected at all.'

This statement was so startling that I asked him to repeat it. I hadn't misheard: despite three consecutive weeks of the most negative publicity imaginable, Billingsgate's throughput of farmed Scottish salmon had remained exactly the same. Was this, I asked, an instance of a new syndrome among the public: food scare fatigue?

'No,' said Chris. 'It's the supermarkets. They anticipated a panic so they slashed their prices. A lot of people stopped buying salmon for a bit, but a lot of others saw how cheap it was and bought it for the first time. If anything it's probably given the salmon market a bit of a fillip.'

Smoked salmon was a luxury when I was small – a special treat that appeared at Christmas time or during visits to my grandmother, and that even then was served on small squares of bread and butter with lemon and pepper. It seemed to deserve its reputation as the King of Fish. These days, salmon is served in a salad at Little Chef restaurants as a healthy alternative to burgers, chips and beans. With government encouragement, the British now eat roughly three times as much salmon as they did ten years ago; Europe-wide, consumption of the fish rose by 14 per cent every year in the 1990s. It was disorientating how thoroughly one of the currencies of my youth had been devalued. Chris the Fish thought the public 'understood' about salmon; but after a visit to a Little Chef on the M4 near Newport one weekend – a visit prompted by curiosity rather than any desire to eat there – it seemed to me that they didn't understand at all. The 'allergy advice' on the restaurant's laminated menu included a warning that the smoked salmon salad 'contains fish'.

At my local fishmonger's I noticed that, although wild Scottish salmon was among the most expensive fish sold, the farmed variety was one of the very cheapest. The difference between them was brought home to me by an environmentalist website that featured something called a SalmoFan. Manufactured by the Swiss pharmaceuticals firm Roche, it resembled an interior decorator's paint swatch and showed a range of more than thirty shades of pink. Wild salmon was pink, I learned, because it fed on krill. Farmed salmon lived in cages and was unable to chase krill. The natural flesh colour of farmed salmon was therefore an unappetising and unmarketable shade of grey. The SalmoFan allowed farmers to preselect the flesh colour of their product by adding Roche-manufactured dyes to its feed.

Until recently the additive most commonly used to colour salmon flesh was Canthaxanthin, a biological pigment used by the pharmaceutical industry in products like Bronze EZ, an ointment popular with body-builders wanting a quick and sunless suntan. Unfortunately the pigment was linked to eye defects in children. In 2003, indeed, the European Commission moved to reduce the level of Canthaxanthin permitted in salmon feed by a factor of four. Nevertheless, research in the US showed that consumers believed that darker salmon colours were indicators of higher quality and better taste. In one study they preferred the SalmoFan colour number 33 by a margin of two to one.

Melissa and I saw this primitive selection technique in action on one of our increasingly rare visits to Tesco. We were queuing at the fish counter where both wild and farmed salmon fillets were on sale. The colour difference was marked. Some of it had been pre-cut into manageable portions, marinaded and dressed with dill; some of it bore a label depicting a picturesque Scottish croft, and the information in quaint Gothic lettering that it had been 'traditionally smoked'. The customer in front of us wanted salmon.

'Four fillets please,' he said, pointing at the ruddiest cuts of flesh, before adding: 'It is organic, isn't it?'

The fishmonger, already flipping the fillets onto wax-paper, paused.

'We don't do organic salmon. But I've got wild over there.'

His customer hesitated; we watched him look along the display at the delicate pink wild fish, and back to the farmed variety.

'Nah, there's something wrong with those . . . I'll take these ones.'

When our turn came, Melissa ordered 'two nice, wild, unfarmed mackerel, please', and was rewarded with a complicit smirk from the fishmonger.

The consumer's world was topsy-turvy. As Joe Strummer once sang for The Clash, we were indeed all lost in the supermarket. The messages we received about food were so confusing and contradictory that, like the man buying salmon, we were sometimes forced to fall back on our most basic instincts; yet even these could not be trusted when they could be manipulated by the simple addition of a little red dye. Tinted salmon was more than a ploy in some harmless marketing game. I was convinced that the dangers of chemical contamination were real.

To Melissa's surprise, I began to amass certain health statistics from the media, cutting out snippets from the news-in-brief columns of newspapers, jotting down things I heard on the radio or dashing off in the middle of TV documentaries to find a pen.

Some scientists blamed chemical changes in the West's diet for a dramatic increase in a range of maladies such as Chronic Fatigue Syndrome, hormone-related imbalances, mental illness, even asthma and eczema in children. Some also blamed chemicals for the extraordinary decline in Western male fertility in the last twenty years. In Denmark, a country particularly badly affected, 40 per cent of men now have subnormal sperm counts. There was no agreed explanation for the unprecedented rise in premature puberty among Western girls, nor for the ever-increasing incidence of breast cancer. In fact, all types of cancer: at some point this century the disorder, a minor killer a hundred years ago, was on course to replace heart disease as the whole of the industrialized world's number-one cause of death. In Britain, the incidence of cancer had risen by 50 per cent since the 1970s. The removal of carcinogens from the national food supply ought logically to have been a priority. Yet as Dasani, Sudan 1 and countless other food scares demonstrated, our food was still riddled with them.

As an expectant parent I was especially intrigued by the state of British children's health. Incipient obesity was just one part of the dietary problem. The explosion of new allergies to foods such as peanuts was common knowledge, but I was startled to discover that as many as 40 per cent of schoolchildren were now thought to have at least one allergy, and that childhood allergies had risen tenfold since 1950. I discovered what this meant in practice from my sister, a nursery school headmistress, who told me that for the last two years her staff members had been obliged to carry auto-injecting EpiPens in case of anaphylactic emergency among their young charges.

1950, I observed, was an important statistical watershed for health researchers. Some 20 per cent of schoolchildren, including a nephew of Melissa's, now suffered from eczema – up from 3 per cent in 1950. In the US, cancer now killed one in four people – up from one in five in 1950, despite the decline of smoking in that time. The incidence of testicular cancer among European men had risen sixfold – again, since 1950. It made me wonder what was so special about that date. It was as though the period preceding it had been some sort of pre-lapsarian paradise.

It didn't take long to work out that the middle of the twentieth century was the starting date for the chemical contamination of modern life. The body of an average Western adult, I learned, now contained measurable traces of between 300 and 500 man-made chemicals. Yet in the 1940s the average Westerner contained no man-made chemicals for the simple reason that those chemicals did not yet exist. In a recent survey conducted by the World Wildlife Fund, volunteers in thirteen British cities had their blood tested for the presence of seventy-seven man-made chemicals. Three main groups of chemical were sought: organochlorine pesticides; polychlorinated bi-phenyls or PCBs, once widely used in the household electronics industry; and flame-retardants of the kind commonly used in paints and furniture. The survey was widely reported. Every single one of the volunteers was found to be multiply contaminated.

The individual amounts of the chemicals that the WWF tested for were mostly tiny and, by themselves, probably harmless. The snag, as Drummond himself pointed out over half a century ago, was that no-one was able to say what might happen to those chemicals once they accumulated and combined over time with others in the body. Biochemists called this unknown consequence the 'cocktail effect'. There were literally billions of possible cocktails: far too many for scientists to be able to test. According to the National Toxicology Program in America, an abbreviated, single-species, thirteen-week toxicity evaluation of all the interactions in a mixture of just twenty-five chemicals would require over 33 million experiments at a cost of about $3 trillion. Not for nothing had one distinguished biochemist described our twentieth-century submersion in chemicals as 'a totally uncontrolled experiment on the human race'.

Chemical poisons could be inhaled, or absorbed through the skin. Sodium laurel sulphate, for instance, a foaming agent frequently used in shampoos and washing-up liquid, had the potential to become carcinogenic when mixed with certain other household chemical products. But the primary route into the human body was ingestion. There were an estimated 3000 chemical food additives and hundreds of pesticides and herbicides in everyday use in the West. The advocates of the organic food movement were surely right to argue that chemicals in the food chain were more responsible for the West's bodily contamination than any other source.

The introduction of new agrochemicals and farming techniques in the 1940s and 1950s led to an extraordinary cultural shift in the way that food was produced. Agrochemicals meant that farmers could grow more food, of course, but the greater significance was that, for the first time, their harvests could virtually be guaranteed. Until the 1940s, growing food had been a risky affair. A crop could be wiped out at any time by blight or aphids or some other accident of nature. With this threat removed by agrochemicals, all that changed. Crop production stabilized, prices dropped – and our relationship with food and the way it was produced was altered for ever. Perhaps for the first time in history, quantity and the price of food became more important than quality. All Western food production was affected, not just crops. The health, size and growth-rate of livestock could also be manipulated by adding antibiotics, hormones and other new compounds to their ever more artificial diet. Farming had become pharming, and 'agrobusiness' was born.

It was easy to condemn the breaking of the ancient bond between man and nature, or to decry the apparently callous industrialization of the countryside. Our home-delivery organics box contained some shocking new fact or other about agrobusiness every week. It was propaganda, and I didn't much like it. I was reminded of the jokes you get in crackers, except that the slips of paper these titbits of information were printed on were always green, and carried a pious assurance that they were the product of '100% sustainable forestry'.

It seemed to me that the box-deliverers were forgetting the context in which agrochemicals were born. Europe had suffered widespread hunger and supply-disruption during six long years of blood-letting and destruction. Farming for the masses was not initiated in the interests of profit. The primary motivation was philanthropic. On the other hand, there seemed little doubt that the cheap and plentiful food the philanthropists were aiming for had led, directly and indirectly, to an unprecedented new dietary crisis. Obesity was merely its most visible symptom. The brave agricultural experiment of the post-war years had run out of control.

Obesity was not a health issue for me and Melissa, but some of the other consequences of the agrochemical revolution were inescapable. One of the most troubling was the nutritive difference between the intensively grown fruits and vegetables of today and their equivalents of sixty years ago. Changes in farming practice had been matched by equally dramatic changes in the food that the farmers produced. According to the government's own data, between 1940 and 1991 the typical British potato 'lost' 47 per cent of its copper, and 45 per cent of its iron. Carrots lost 75 per cent of their magnesium, and broccoli 75 per cent of its calcium. The pattern was repeated for vitamins. A study in Canada showed that between 1951 and 1999, potatoes lost all of their vitamin A and 57 per cent of their vitamin C, while today's consumers would have to eat as many as eight oranges to obtain the same amount of vitamin A as their grandparents did from a single fruit.

I had always assumed that eating healthily was a simple matter of cutting out junk food and following the government's much publicized advice to eat five portions of fruit and vegetables a day. At least 700 food brands in the UK used the government's five-a-day logo on their packaging. But if the 'healthy' option was literally no longer what it used to be, what did the government's programme – which enjoyed the endorsement of the World Health Organization – really mean? Any amount of fruit and veg was better than none, of course. It was sensible to promote it in a country where a fifth of teenagers ate no fruit at all. But it was still unclear how the government defined an orange. Organic, or intensively grown? What vintage was it measuring? Had it taken nutrient depletion into account? What, precisely, were we supposed to be eating five a day of?

It was much the same with chicken. In 1976 the public were officially encouraged by the Royal College of Physicians to eat less red meat, which is high in heart-attack-inducing saturated fats, and to switch to lean white meat instead. As a result, British consumption of chicken doubled to around 30 kg per person per year. Chicken was still perceived, marketed and promoted by the FSA as a 'healthy' food. (For extra healthiness, the FSA recommended removing its skin.) But since the 1970s, chicken itself had changed. Modern battery chickens, I learned, were so intensively reared that they were sometimes brought to market in as little as five weeks from the egg. They grew so fast that they had no time to put on much muscle tissue; they were so busy eating that they took little exercise. They were, essentially, obese animals: according to one study, a modern supermarket bird contained twice as much fat as its equivalent in 1940, even without its skin. All that fat had to go somewhere. Fat chickens meant fat people. I was ten in 1976 and remember eating chicken then. In our family we ate it once week at most, usually for Sunday lunch, because in those days it was expensive as well as lean. Thirty years later, Asda was selling a family-sized chicken for just over £2. It was there for all to see: in one generation a health food had effectively become a junk food, just as salmon had.

My fascination with the food chain was deepening fast. One day I marched into the kitchen where Melissa was busy with our Russell Hobbs bread-maker (a wedding present that she actually used).

'This agrobusiness business is pernicious!' I said, waving a newspaper cutting. 'Do you realize how much milk a modern dairy cow produces compared to 1956? Go on, guess.'

Melissa looked at me with one eyebrow raised, and said nothing. It was a look she had given me quite often in recent days.

'OK, I'll tell you anyway. It's 9000 kilos a year when it used to be 2000. How can that be right? It's a perversion of nature!'

'James,' Melissa said. 'Do you think you might be going a little bit mad?'

'No – why?'

'Because if anyone's in danger of becoming an orthorexic these days it's not me, it's you.'

'I didn't say I was going to stop putting milk in my tea. I only meant that it's rather shocking to find out how it's produced.'

'I know, darling,' she said, kissing me on the cheek, 'but it's important to keep a sense of proportion about these things. It's only milk you're talking about, and it's enough that the milk in our fridge already comes in a carton that says "organic". OK?'

She was right. I was starting to resemble 'K', the hypochondriac hero of Jerome K. Jerome's 1889 classic *Three Men in a Boat*, who went one day to the British Library to look up the symptoms of hay fever in a medical dictionary. 'And then, in an unthinking moment, I idly turned the leaves, and began indolently to study diseases, generally ... I plodded conscientiously through the twenty-six letters, and the only malady I could conclude I had not got was housemaid's knee ... I walked into that reading-room a happy healthy man. I crawled out a decrepit wreck.' Nutrition was an inexact science; a little knowledge could be a dangerous thing. As Melissa said, it was important to keep a sense of proportion. Common sense had to be applied. Yet I was still troubled by the super-cows, and the milk jetting through their udders so many times faster than God intended. How could there not be a nutritional price to pay for such flagrant tampering with nature?

I looked into it. This time, I didn't share my findings with Melissa. A new study of government figures by the nutritionist David Thomas found that between 1940 and 2000 British milk had lost 2 per cent of its calcium, 21 per cent of its magnesium and 60 per cent of its iron. The figures for certain cheeses were even worse. Parmesan, for instance, had lost 70 per cent of its magnesium, while its iron content had disappeared altogether. The figures were naturally disputed. The FSA, with weary predictability, argued that historical comparisons were worthless because of 'differences in analytical methodology'. This was despite confirmation from within the dairy industry that David Thomas was right. 'Our methods of making cheese have not changed, but milk in 1940 was not the same as milk today,' said Leo Bertozzi, the director of the Italian parmesan consortium. 'Today cows yield five to six times as many litres a day, and their feed is different, with cereals and soya added to hay.' The grass that modern cows ate was different, too. Gillian Butler, a researcher at the University of Newcastle, put it very simply: 'The faster grass grows, the more the uptake of trace elements is diluted.'

There were sound reasons and powerful arguments for the post-war industrialization of agriculture. Perhaps nutrient depletion was a price worth paying for the advantages of having enough food. Yet the chemical interference with our diet that accompanied industrialization was not inevitable. Jack Drummond sounded a note of caution as early as 1927, when he sent a letter to *The Times* in which he attacked the German practice of irradiating children's milk. 'Milk which has been exposed to the radiations of a mercury-vapour lamp . . . suffers chemical changes which are highly undesirable from the standpoint of nutrition,' he wrote. 'The tendency to apply somewhat generally the results of laboratory research before they are ripe for practical use is to be regretted.'

It was only a few months since Melissa and I had started taking delivery of an organic groceries box. The overflowing fruit-bowl on our kitchen table made me feel downright smug at first, but now I looked at it with a jaundiced eye. It seemed sad – tragic, even – that we had been reduced to such a measure. It was surely reasonable to expect ordinary food to be free of body-polluting chemicals, and for dietary staples to be as nutritious as they had been for thousands of years before 1950. In a sane world there would be no need for organic food, and the billion-pound industry of which we had become a part would not exist. The organic milk in our fridge and the fruit-bowl on our table signified that somehow, somewhere, the West had taken a disastrous wrong turn.

Chapter 3

The Agrochemical Revolution

'The Federal Drug Administration of the USA has a list of 800 chemicals now in use, or proposed for use, in foods. The list is growing rapidly. With each addition the chemist's responsibility to the consuming public increases. It is a simple matter to ascertain whether the new chemical compounds are active poisons, but it is much more difficult to answer with assurance the question whether these substances will have harmful effects on health if they are taken in to the body in small quantities over periods of years.'

Jack Drummond, *Chemistry and Food* lecture (1951)

Melissa's clothes no longer fitted her. She wrapped her party dresses in plastic, put them on hangers at the back of the bedroom cupboard, and went out to shop for jeans with elasticated waistbands and extra-large bras. My mother knitted a tiny sweater. My sister produced an old wooden cradle that she no longer needed. I bought a second-hand pram on e-Bay from someone in Newcastle, and felt self-satisfied about the money I'd saved on a new one from Mothercare. Domestication crept up on us like a mugger in the park. In between times I plunged back into Drummond's post-war world.

Unlike the world-shaking events of the 1940s or the sexual and cultural revolution of the 1960s, the early 1950s was not a period of British history that had much interested me before. I tended to think of it in clichés: a Routemaster bus picking its way through the London smog; the coronation of Elizabeth II and the conquest of Everest; Roger Bannister and the four-minute mile. But despite these iconic images, the adjective I most associated with the decade was 'drab'. I was not alone: when I entered 'drab' and '1950s' on my computer's search engine, it returned over 9000 results. The stereotype was wrong, of course. The post-war period was a time of profound change that still shapes the modern world. The independence of Israel was recognized in 1948, engendering a conflict that continues to consume the Middle East; Monnet, Schuman and Adenauer laid the foundations of European Union in 1950; the Cold War crystallized, setting a bi-polar political agenda in the West that lasted for forty years and has still not been fully supplanted.

The troops returning to Britain in their hundreds of thousands from combat had the highest expectations of the peace. Imbued with the spirit of 'never again', they were looking for nothing less than a new order in the nation they had fought to defend; and in 1945, to the astonishment of Winston Churchill and the Conservative Party, they voted for one. Clement Attlee's Labour government came to power with the stated intention of establishing the 'Socialist Commonwealth of Great Britain', a new utopia that would be 'free, democratic, efficient, progressive, public-spirited, its material resources organized in the service of the British people'.

Of the many issues facing the country, domestic food supply was perhaps the most pressing. No-one could forget how malnutrition had blighted life in the cities during the economic depression before the war. Politically, a return to the social conditions of the 1930s had to be avoided at all costs. For this reason, 'Agriculture and the People's Food' enjoyed a section of its own in Attlee's manifesto. 'Agriculture is not only a job for the farmers; it is also a way of feeding the people. So . . . our agriculture should be planned to give us the food we can best produce at home, and large enough to give us as much of those foods as possible . . . The people need food at prices they can afford to pay. This means that our food supplies will have to be planned.'

Food planning: this was what Jack Drummond had been all about. Attlee was specific in his acknowledgement of Drummond's wartime contribution. 'The Ministry of Food has done fine work for the housewife in war,' the manifesto said. 'The Labour Party intends to keep going as much of the work of the Ministry of Food as will be useful in peace conditions ... A Labour Government will keep the new food services, such as the factory canteens and British restaurants, free and cheap milk for mothers and children, fruit juices and food supplements, and will improve and extend these services.'

In theory, no-one was better placed to oversee the running of these popular services than their architect: the new knight of the people, Sir Jack Drummond. No-one else bridged the gap between academia and Whitehall quite so effectively, nor possessed the lightness of touch with which to exploit that position. For a nutritionist as philanthropic as Drummond, the election of a government as populist as Attlee's should have been the best possible news – an opportunity to defend and extend the advances in public nutrition made during the war, and even to influence the future direction of agricultural policy.

In practice, the upheaval in the House of Commons passed Drummond by. In 1944 he was appointed an adviser on nutrition to SHAEF, the Supreme Headquarters, Allied Expeditionary Force. Although he was officially seconded to the Ministry of Food until 1946, for the next two years he was more often on the continent than at home. At the time of Attlee's victory at the polls, and for several months afterwards, he was to be found in Germany and Austria, working for the new Allied Control Commissions, whose job was to restore a semblance of order to the shattered Reich. He was therefore out of the country and out of the loop during the new government's crucial early period. Nor was there anyone in London to represent his interests, or to suggest that a senior peacetime role might usefully be found for him within the administration. Drummond's best political contact was his friend and former employer, the Minister of Food, Lord Woolton; but Woolton, one of Churchill's closest allies, was a Tory, and the Tories were now out in the cold. In short, circumstances combined to ensure that Drummond missed the moment. Released from his duties on the continent, he returned home to a directorship at the Boots Pure Drug Company in Nottingham, a sinecure far from the centre of power.

No doubt he was pleased that the new government planned to go on supplying schoolchildren with free milk – although the motivation for their doing so had changed. During the war such services had been introduced as a survival tactic. Now, with the U-boats beaten and the sea lanes open again, they were to be continued for ideological reasons. If the public thought the peace dividend was to include an end to rationing, they were to be sorely disappointed. Rationing got worse before it got better after the war, and didn't end fully until 1954, fifteen years after it began.

The war had been financially ruinous: 28 per cent of the country's wealth had been wiped out, twice as much as in 1914–18. The Lend-Lease agreement with America that had underpinned the economy for years was abruptly terminated by President Truman when the Japanese surrendered. And yet the uncomfortable fact of economic dependence on America took a long time to sink in. Britain was not ready to give up its image of itself as a Great Power, and persisted in behaving like one. Defence spending accounted for 18 per cent of GNP in 1948, when a million men were still under arms. Troop levels were maintained by the introduction of National Service in 1947. The new recruits were deployed in many places, although the great majority were sent to police the British zone of occupied Germany. The main reason for the rationing of bread in 1947–8 – something that had not happened even in the darkest days of the war – was the obligation to feed the starving German population. No-one had dreamed that victory could taste so bitter.

The public naturally grumbled. Some blamed the Opposition. Attlee had been elected by a nation eager to reject the aristocratic old order, whose policies were perceived to have led the country into not one but two disastrous world wars. The Right and the profligate rich were therefore an easy target for the far Left. 'Today, the great hotels and the expensive City restaurants are packed to the door with people eating as well as they ever ate in their lives,' a Scottish Communist Party pamphlet frothed in 1946. 'There is no control at all in the private rooms of hotels and the homes of the rich, and every food racketeer and black market scoundrel can find ready customers for everything they can lay illegal hands on . . . More than anyone else, the traditional enemies of the working class, the Tory Party, are responsible for the food crisis.' But the Tories were not really responsible. With the notable exception of America, all countries suffered food shortages after the war, not just Britain. The entire world was exhausted, and Attlee's government was too broke to buy its way out of trouble.

The masses were not to be denied, however. Only one solution presented itself: Britain would have to produce yet more of its own food. And that is what happened: between 1947 and 1951 the value of farm industry output doubled to £1bn, a figure that exceeded the government's most optimistic forecast for 1951 by a factor of five. Production in sectors such as animal husbandry rose even more spectacularly. Pork production rose from 11,000 tons in 1947 to 241,000 tons in 1953.

Rapid mechanization played a critical role in the agricultural explosion. The number of tractors on British farms rose from 101,500 in 1942 to 324,960 in 1952. The number of combine harvesters and potato diggers rose sixteenfold over the same period, while hay balers, grain driers and milking machines were introduced for the first time. The transformation prompted the young Duke of Edinburgh to joke at a farmers' dinner: 'We now need a machine to help us decide which machine to buy.' Yet mechanization was only a part of the story. At least as significant – and from the modern health perspective, more so – was the first mass-application of fertilizer, weed-killer and pesticides to the land. Fertilizer prices had been subsidized by the government during the war, a policy that was not discontinued after it. British farmers had spent about £8m on fertilizer in 1939. By 1947 they were spending £33m, and by 1953, £66m.

Drummond did not disapprove of artificial fertilizers. He was not a Luddite, but a modern man of science who believed that the solution to the world's food shortage could well be chemical. In 1951 he gave a carefully reasoned lecture entitled *Chemistry and Food* under the auspices of the prestigious Chemical Council; the text of his lecture was published posthumously the following year. In it, he sang the praises of John Bennett Lawes, whose nineteenth-century experiments with bone ash on a farm at Rothamsted were 'the birth of the great artificial fertilizer industry'. According to a recent United Nations report, he pointed out with evident enthusiasm, 'supplies of most fertilizers have become sufficient to meet effective world demand for the first time since the war'. World supply in 1951 amounted to some 13 million tons, fully a fifth of which was produced in Britain.

Even in 1951 there were those who worried that crops grown in chemically treated soil could be deficient in nutrients. Drummond, I was slightly surprised to discover, was dismissive of the theory. 'There is much to appeal to the imagination in the view, not infrequently expressed by some agriculturists, that a purely chemical approach to the problem of fertility of the soil must inevitably lead to crops becoming less nutritious to man and livestock,' he told his Chemical Council audience. 'Intriguing as this theory may be, up to now no scientific evidence has been produced to support it.'

Such breezy scepticism was typical of him; it was also solidly in tune with the times. Several decades were to pass before the emergence of evidence linking nutrient depletion to intensive farming methods.

Where other agrochemicals were concerned, however, Drummond was far more visionary. 'In countless laboratories the world over,' he said in the same lecture, 'chemists are striving to produce compounds that will prove to be effective insecticides, potent fungicides, poisons for pests such as rats, or drugs to combat animal diseases. These are formidable tasks. They would be easier if we had better comprehension of the relation between the chemical structure of a compound and its biological action. Unfortunately, extensive study of this relationship has revealed many more anomalies than ordered patterns. That being so, there is nothing for it but to submit each new compound to a wide range of tests so as to ascertain its action not only on the parasite or micro-organism it is desired to kill, but on the host organism as well.'

The government, unfortunately, wasn't interested in testing for 'anomalies'. Their priority was more and cheaper food, and the new generation of agrochemicals produced fabulous results. The average per-acre crop yield for barley rose by 45 per cent between 1940 and 1955. Wheat rose by 43 per cent, sugar beet by 37 per cent, and corn by 29 per cent. Chemicals could help to preserve stocks as well as increase harvests. The loss of stored cereals to rodents and grain pests such as weevil, for instance, had been a serious problem during the war. In 1943 the amount of grain lost in this way was said to have exceeded the tonnage claimed by U-boats. There was little the authorities could do about this then, but post-war advances in the laboratories meant that such vast losses were soon a thing of the past.

One evening, as I was reading about one of those advances – the 1948 introduction to the market of Warfarin, the first ever target-specific rodenticide and a milestone in the war on rats – I heard a piercing scream from the kitchen. I hurried downstairs to find Melissa backed away from the bread-making machine.

'I can't believe it. There's a . . . *beast* in there,' she said. 'Will you deal with it? Please?'

The top of the machine was closed. I took up a carving knife and, with my arm fully extended, inserted the tip beneath the lid and flipped it open, deftly springing back at the same time.

'No, not in there . . . *there*,' she wailed, stabbing a finger at the little LCD clock that flashed to let you know when the bread was baked. 'God, it's huge.'

I peered cautiously at the screen. Trapped between the clock and the glass that covered it was a wriggling maggot.

'Hmm,' I said. 'That flour you've been using is organic, isn't it?'

In 1949, I had just read, Attlee's government had passed the Prevention of Damage by Pests Act, a piece of legislation that was still on the statute books. The Act made the use of pesticides on farms obligatory in certain circumstances. Now I thought I could see why.

'We'll have to throw the whole thing away,' said Melissa.

'What? You can't do that, it's almost new!'

'I *can't* eat maggots.'

'It's the flour you need to chuck out. I can clean the bread-maker.'

I took the motherboard apart with a Phillips screwdriver. There were only two maggots inside, one of them already dead. In any case, by the time I had finished I had changed my mind about where they had come from: a fly had probably got in via a small vent-hole at the back, and its eggs had hatched in the warmth of the electronic circuitry. There was no accounting for the strength of Melissa's reaction. Despite routinely brushing bugs and manure from the vegetables in our delivery box, the larva stage of *Musca domestica* was too much for her. I convinced her in the end not to banish the bread-maker, although it was weeks before she bought flour again. Just as in 1942 when Drummond altered the B-vitamin content of the national loaf, domestic confidence in wholemeal bread had temporarily collapsed.

The scientists of the post-war period enjoyed the specific blessing of government. There was a widespread acknowledgement that British ingenuity, represented by that endearing and enduring stereotype, the backroom boffin, had contributed enormously to the victory of 1945. The battle for air supremacy over the south coast in 1940 wouldn't have been won without radar and the Spitfire. Innovations in ordnance by men like Barnes Wallis, the inventor of the bouncing bomb, played a critical role in the weakening of Nazi Germany. The atomic bomb drops on Japan shortened the war in the East and arguably saved hundreds of thousands of Allied lives. Immediately after the war, therefore, it was natural that scientists should be seen as the standard-bearers of a brave new world, who would transform the misery of the 1940s into a bright and glorious future.

'The Labour Party intends to link the skill of British craftsmen and designers to the skill of British scientists in the service of our fellow men,' Attlee's manifesto stated. 'The genius of British scientists and technicians, who have produced radio-location, jet propulsion, penicillin and the Mulberry Harbours in wartime, must be given full rein in peacetime too.'

The legislation brought forward during the Attlee years was typically based not on the findings of focus-groups or even on socialist ideology, but on hard, scientific evidence. For statisticians, these were the glory days. An army of bowler-hatted civil servants rose to prominence at the heart of government and brought new meaning to the term 'central control'. The extent of official influence over daily life fifty years ago would probably be considered intrusive today – or else just plain absurd. An item I spotted in a 1952 issue of the *Chemistry and Industry Journal* neatly illustrated the period's touching faith in the power of science, even if it now reads like source material for a sketch by Monty Python:

> ❧ ⌁
>
> ### SAFETY FOOTWEAR
>
> In 1950 the number of foot injuries in industry amounted to 29,000 in the UK. Of these, between 12,000 and 15,000 came within the category of 'factory accidents', as distinct from mining, railway and other non-factory industrial accidents. These figures were given to Mr Harold Watkinson MP, Parliamentary Secretary to the Ministry of Labour, at a Press conference on 'Safety Footwear' held in London on September 9. The occasion was the introduction of a new British Standard 'Men's Safety Boots and Shoes' (B.S.1870:1952), which specifies minimum requirements for safety boots and shoes provided with protective steel toecaps.

After the conference a practical test of the footwear was arranged.
Mr George Denton, Chairman of the British Standards Institution
Committee on Safety Footwear, wearing the protective shoes,
allowed a standard double-decker London bus to run over
the toe of one of his shoes.

ở ↗

The 'full rein' that Attlee granted to 'the genius of British scientists' sent a clear signal to the agrochemists. They had effectively been given carte blanche to develop whatever it took to increase home food production, and they duly went to work. Between 1945 and 1950, twenty new agrochemical companies entered the world market. They were more successful than they could ever have anticipated: worldwide sales of agrochemicals grew by 7 per cent every year between 1945 and 1960. By the 1990s, the total world market in agrochemicals was worth more than $21bn.

The leader of the British pack was Imperial Chemical Industries. They were responsible for one of the most important agrochemicals of the post-war period, although it had actually been discovered earlier, in 1940. An ICI scientist called Bill Templeman observed that when a natural plant hormone called alpha-naphthylacetic acid, or NAA, was ploughed into the soil, it killed yellow charlock without affecting the oats that were also growing there. This led to the development of the world's first selective hormone weed-killer: 4-chloro-2-methylphenoxyacetic acid, or MCPA.

The development history of MCPA makes alarming reading today. Public health and safety was clearly not much of a concern for the specialists whose job it was to assess the new compound. In December 1942 Robert Hudson, the Minister of Agriculture, held a meeting with Templeman and several senior ICI executives, and agreed to the setting up of 300 MCPA testing centres around the country. The operation was supposed to be a secret, because the new compound was deemed even then to have great military potential – as a defoliant, for example. In practice, the field trials were more like an episode from *Keystone Cops*. 'Mobile teams toured the country in specially equipped lorries, and tests were carried out on hundreds of different soils and crops, all in the utmost secrecy because of wartime security', according to one account. 'This occasionally led to all sorts of excitement as the suspicions of country policemen were aroused by the sinister appearance of shrouded lorries, or when a sudden change in the wind blew the dust into someone's prized garden.'

By 1947 'Cornland Cleaner', as MCPA was branded, was one of ICI's best-sellers – the progenitor of the so-called 'phenoxy' family of herbicides which formed the bedrock of an extraordinary weed-killer revolution. There had been a limited amount of crop-spraying with weed-killer before the war, when horse-drawn carts spread a primitive substance made from diluted sulphuric acid. Post-war, crop-spraying was as rapidly mechanized as everything else: between 1942 and 1952 the number of mechanical crop-sprayers on farms in England and Wales rose from 4750 to 17,340. A dozen companies specialized in the new machinery. Innovations in spraying technology were frequently underwritten by the chemical manufacturers themselves. The mid-1940s 'Agro-Sprayer', for instance, was manufactured by Ransomes under licence from Plant Protection Ltd, a subsidiary of ICI. It worked by atomizing the chemical and distributing it under air pressure through a jet nozzle, which was far more efficient and cost-effective than earlier methods.

In 1942, in the interests of secrecy, the government forbade ICI to file for foreign patents for MCPA. The gesture proved futile when the new compound's action was described in an American magazine article. The Americans soon developed their own NAA-based compound: 2,4-dichlorophenoxyacetic acid, or 2,4-D. The British had been right to try to keep the new technology under wraps, for it did indeed have military potential: in the 1960s, 2,4-D became one of the two main ingredients of Agent Orange, the most infamous military defoliant in history. Between

1965 and 1971 the US air force sprayed some 20 million gallons of Agent Orange – and its lesser-known cousins Agents White, Blue, Purple, Pink and Green – over Vietnam.

ICI and its rivals showed little interest in investigating the potential effects of their products on human health. It would be many years before even the environmental side-effects of mass-crop-spraying were properly noticed by the public, with the 1962 publication of Rachel Carson's ground-breaking polemic *Silent Spring*. The carelessness with which the agrochemists proceeded seems incredible today, when the carcinogenic or mutagenetic effects of many of the phenoxy herbicides are beyond dispute. Agent Orange is a case in point. The substance was used to deprive the enemy of cover, but also to clear foliage behind the American lines – along roadsides, for instance, or around the perimeters of jungle camps. The US servicemen and women on whom it rained were specifically told that it was harmless. Some of the pilots of the specialist C-123 tanker planes are even reputed to have drunk it, as part of a squadron initiation rite. Agent Orange was later found to contain Dioxin, and linked to cancer and behavioral disorders in veterans as well as birth abnormalities in their children. A million people are still estimated to be affected. Dioxin levels in the lake that supplies the inhabitants of the town of Bien Hoa, once the US air force HQ in Vietnam, are still 200 times the WHO's recommended maximum. In Ho Chi Minh City a baby with a birth defect continues to be born every other day.

I could understand why the precautionary principle might not have counted for much among scientific researchers in the crisis years of the 1940s. On the other hand, not everyone was sanguine about the risks of agrochemicals, even in the early days. One notable opponent was Eve Balfour, whose 1943 book *The Living Soil* presented the case for farming without chemicals – an approach she pioneered at New Bells Farm in Suffolk, and which today is called organic farming. She was influenced by, among others, Sir Robert McCarrison, a former Indian army medical officer whose extensive research had demonstrated the link between disease in industrial societies and diets made defective by food processing. He was especially critical of the use of chemical additives as a substitute for fresh food. Publication of *The Living Soil* led directly to the foundation in 1946 of the Soil Association, whose purpose was to highlight the connection between farming practice and plant, animal, human and environmental health, and to promote organic agriculture as a sustainable alternative to intensive farming methods. Eve Balfour was dismissed as a crank by most of her contemporaries. She was, of course, years ahead of her time. Today the Soil Association is the principal certifying authority of the organic food industry; Sainsbury's even sell a breed of potato that is named after her.

The other opponent was Jack Drummond. He did not agree with Eve Balfour about the use of fertilizers, but where the use of herbicides and pesticides were concerned they spoke with a very similar voice. By 1952, 'anomalies' in the biological behaviour of new chemicals that he had warned about in his lecture to the Chemical Council were popping up all over the place. The behaviour of Dichlorodiphenyltrichloroethane – better known as DDT – was a case in point. The insecticidal properties of this famous compound, the first of a new class of pesticide called the organochlorines, were discovered by the chemist Paul Müller of the Swiss firm Geigy in 1939. As the fight with Germany turned into a proper world war, troops were increasingly deployed in jungle theatres where malaria-carrying mosquitoes were often as dangerous as the enemy. DDT was first used in combat in 1943 by the US army, and the British soon copied them.

In 1951, Drummond reported that American studies had found traces of DDT in milk intended for human consumption (DDT was much used in dairies to destroy flies). The human health consequences of this migration, he advised, were still unknown. 'There is no doubting that remarkable benefits to mankind have accrued from the use of this one chemical, but the chemist is now faced by a variety of further problems as a direct outcome of his own efforts,' he warned.

There was another DDT anomaly that frightened Drummond: the

emergence of insects with the ability to resist it. This unexpected phenomenon was first observed in Italy as early as 1947. By 1952, when DDT-resistance had spread everywhere from Russia to California, the anomaly had become a pattern. This, perhaps, was the true cost of the Attlee policy of giving peacetime scientists 'full rein'. The folly of ignoring the precautionary principle, and of not thoroughly testing new products before rushing them to market, was becoming increasingly clear. If nature could evolve resistance to DDT, Drummond reasoned, the same thing was likely to happen with other chemicals. His prediction was accurate. Today, more than 500 insect species are known to be resistant to at least one formulation of insecticide; at least seventeen species are resistant to all major classes of insecticide. It is the same story in the plant world, where eighty-four species of weed are now able to resist herbicides. There are even five kinds of rat known to be resistant to the chemicals used against them.

The environmental degradation DDT caused is a matter of record. DDT sprayed on crops in the US affected the diet of wild birds so badly that the shells of the eggs they laid were catastrophically thinned; in the 1960s, America's national symbol, the bald-headed eagle, was driven to the point of extinction. The risk posed by DDT to human health is still disputed, although a link to various forms of cancer and serious reproductive problems has long been suspected; it was finally banned in Britain in 1984. The American anarchist Murray Bookchin, a beret-wearing icon of the 1960s, put it nicely: 'It would seem to be a form of ecological retribution that the very forces man has summoned against the living world around him are being redirected by a remorseless logic against the human organism itself.'

The Minister of Agriculture responsible for persuading the nation's farmers to switch to the new chemicals was Tom Williams, later Lord Williams of Barnburgh, one of Attlee's closest allies. An ex-coalminer from Derbyshire, Williams had no experience of farming. The same was true of Percy Collick, his deputy, who was a former train driver. The jacket of Williams's 1965 autobiography, *Digging for Britain*, depicts the pitheads and slagheap of a coalmine, the view partially obscured by a tangle of wheat stalks in the foreground. A new industrial era in agriculture had begun.

Williams's strategy was as simple as it was successful. First, he offered farmers a fixed and guaranteed price for the staple products that the country most badly needed. 'It had always been my Party's contention that wildly fluctuating prices made it impossible for the British farmer to plan ahead with breeding, cultivation or anything else,' he wrote. Price guarantees removed the greatest financial risk faced by farmers, while offering them an incentive to produce as much as possible.

Secondly, he could wield a big stick if this carrot didn't work. Under the 1947 Agricultural Act, farmers were obliged to follow 'the rules of good estate management and good husbandry' in order to maintain 'a reasonable standard of efficient production, as respects both the kind of produce and the quality and quantity thereof'. What constituted good estate management and efficient production was, of course, decided by the Ministry of Agriculture. If, in the judgement of the Ministry's inspectors, a farm was failing to fulfil its productive potential, it could be placed under state 'supervision'. And if that didn't scare the farmer into compliance, the state ultimately had the right to expropriate his farm. It was perhaps the closest Britain ever came to Stalinism.

ھ ‎ ‎ ‎ ‎

10 & 11 GEO.6. Agriculture Act, 1947

Ch. 48.

Dispossession of owners or occupiers on grounds of
bad estate management or bad husbandry.

Part II. – cont.

16. – (I) Where a supervision order is in force in relation to the
management of the land, and the Minister is satisfied that
the management thereof does not while the order is in force show

satisfactory improvement, and certifies accordingly, the Minister
shall subject to the provisions of this section have power to
purchase compulsorily in accordance with the provisions of
this Act in that behalf the land to which the order relates
or any part of that land.

๛ ๛

This was no idle threat. Between 1948 and 1952 some 4000 supervision orders were issued, and more than 250 farmers and landowners were dispossessed. The definition of 'good estate management' now officially included the use of approved agrochemicals such as MCPA. The government's power to force farmers to use pesticides was further strengthened in 1949, with the passing of the Prevention of Damage by Pests Act. After 1947 Eve Balfour, busily pioneering an alternative approach to agriculture, was probably lucky that the government didn't expropriate her Suffolk farm.

But on the whole, few farmers protested at the new arrangements. The financial incentive on offer from the Ministry was substantial, and farmers were given every encouragement to take it. A National Agricultural Advisory Service was inaugurated in 1946. Some 1400 technical officers were employed to roam the countryside, offering farmers free advice on how to translate the latest scientific advances into useful reality. Some farmers no doubt carped that to take this advice was obligatory. But overall, and certainly compared to the 1930s, there had never been a better time to be in farming.

'I can't believe the government could have been so stupid,' said Melissa from the sofa. 'Didn't they stop to think what spraying chemicals on everything in sight might do to people?'

She was so pregnant now that she could only lie comfortably on her back. Her maternity leave was due to start soon; she looked like the snake that swallowed an elephant in the opening pages of Saint-Exupéry's *The Little Prince*.

'Poor Eugenie,' she went on. 'It just makes me so cross.'

This was a reference to her aunt, who for the last two years had been in the grip of a degenerative brain disorder called Progressive Supranuclear Palsy, a rapacious and heart-rending condition that afflicted, and eventually killed, the comedian Dudley Moore. Vivacious and witty by nature, she had completely lost the ability to speak in recent months, and was increasingly immobile. Her doctors were unable to say what caused her PSP, but it was her conviction that the spraying of pesticides in fields around her home in Wiltshire in the late 1970s was responsible.

It was not until 1950 that Attlee's administration began to have any misgivings about the agrochemical revolution that it had done so much to encourage. A Ministry of Agriculture committee was convened in that year to examine whether the chemicals the public was increasingly exposed to might be detrimental to their health. It was the first time that officialdom had even hinted that there might be such a downside to Tom Williams's policies – although by 1950 it was probably already too late. Even at this early stage, the variety of interests vested in the new industry was so wide that the committee hearings lasted for two years. The agrochemical cat was already out of the bag.

The evidence heard by the committee was conflicting and inconclusive. The human health effects even of DDT were still unknown. The final result was a terrible cop-out. The committee's main recommendation was the setting up of another committee, a body of experts whose task would be to 'advise generally' on problems relating to consumer health. The experts' remit did include 'guiding departments in the investigations which manufacturers would be obliged to make before new chemical products were licensed'. For cost reasons, however, there was no recommendation that the safety of new agrochemicals should be tested independently.

The 1950 committee was chaired by Sir Solly Zuckerman, a zoologist by training who knew little about agrochemicals and expressed surprise at his initial appointment. In a chapter of his autobiography candidly entitled 'An Amateur in Whitehall', Zuckerman wrote: 'We had several discussions about the desirability of compulsory and statutory controls, but in the end decided that a voluntary arrangement with the industries concerned was the best that was then possible.' With that decision, ultimate responsibility for assessing the human health risk of agro-chemicals was left up to the manufacturers for the next thirty years. Statutory controls were not introduced in place of Zuckerman's 'voluntary arrangement' until October 1986. An important opportunity to apply the brakes had been missed.

Another committee, convened in 1953 to examine the effect of agrochemicals on wildlife, was equally ineffective. The field trials it conducted lasted two years, yet were scandalously under-funded. Just 120 acres of wheat and Brussels sprouts in Norfolk and Gloucestershire were examined, at a time when 2.6 million acres of farmland were already under chemical treatment. Moreover, the study focused on the effects of just one agrochemical, a German-invented organophosphate called Schradan, whose indiscriminate deadliness was so obvious that most farmers had already stopped using it of their own accord. In 1952 a 46-acre field of Schradan-treated Brussels sprouts near Charlton Abbots was found to contain the corpses of the following fauna:

Partridges	19
Pheasants	10
Wild birds, various (blackbirds, finches, tits, etc.)	129
Rabbits	7
Hares	2
Rats	2
Mice	4
Grey squirrels	1
Stoats	1
Total corpses found	175

Dramatic as this sounded, it was hardly enough to give a true picture of the situation in the countryside. It was certainly no basis for proposing new legislation. Zuckerman's enquiry ended with a weak recommendation that more research should be done. 'The trouble was that while the profitability of modern agricultural practices could be assessed in monetary terms, the costs of the damage they brought to the countryside could not,' he wrote. 'Protecting the environment was a "social good", and had to find its place in a long list of others.'

Did the government deliberately appoint a self-confessed amateur to the crucial post of pesticides committee chairman? The conspiracy-minded might think so. Zuckerman certainly became a favourite appointee, eventually chairing three separate committees relating to the effects of agrochemicals. To be fair, one of his committees, convened to recommend measures to protect agricultural workers, was an unqualified success. Zuckerman had been impressed by the story of a group of farm labourers who came in from the fields to a local pub and ordered their usual pints of beer. One of them wiped his mouth with the back of his hand and within a few minutes had fallen to the floor, dead. The men had been working with an organophosphate insecticide. In future, they would be obliged by law to wear protective clothing.

Yet worker protection was an easy and obvious target for legislation. Zuckerman's failure to grasp the nettle of regulation elsewhere was abject. He might, for instance, have done more to ensure that the advice he received was impartial. As it was, the make-up of his committees was anything but independent. The seventeen members of his 1953 committee included representatives of ICI, Geigy, and the powerful new Association of British Insecticide Manufacturers. Notable by their absence was anyone who might have advocated restraint.

Such cosiness between government and industry now sounds familiar. Half a century on, a story was rumbling in the press that the Pesticides Safety Directorate, an agency of DEFRA, the Department for the Environment, Food and Rural Affairs, had chosen to ignore the dangers to the public of twenty-first-century pesticides, particularly crop-sprays.

The PSD's advice to DEFRA was supposed to be independent. At the same time, the agency had to achieve 'full cost recovery' for its operations; and the most lucrative part of the PSD's remit, accounting for some 60 per cent of its annual revenue, was the licensing of new agrochemicals. This meant that it collected about £7m a year directly from the agrochemical industry – hardly an arrangement designed to safeguard the independence of the agency's advice.

Michael Meacher, a recently retired Environment Minister, was incensed by the situation. He believed that poisoning by agrochemicals – specifically, of people living in rural areas and inadvertently exposed to crop-sprays – was a far commoner complaint than most people supposed, even in modern-day Britain. Yet the government had neither collated any data nor monitored any side-effects relating to the use of agrochemicals. This allowed the PSD to claim, truthfully, that there was no evidence to support a link between crop-sprays and ill-health and (more controversially) that a robust system was in place to protect the public. 'Will there be the wind of change blowing away the secrecy and complacency involved in licensing these hazardous chemicals,' Meacher wrote in the *Guardian*, 'or will the status quo, so strenuously defended by government and industry, remain?' The status quo, I could see now, was over fifty years old; the *laissez-faire* attitude displayed by Sir Solly Zuckerman had set a standard that had since become institutionalized.

I contacted the Pesticides Action Network, the principal anti-agrochemical lobby group in the UK. Their website asserted that in developing countries, pesticides caused 3 million poisonings and 20,000 deaths every year. I thought it best to ignore this startling claim and to keep my enquiry focused on what was provable, here at home: could they put me in touch with a British victim of pesticide-poisoning? Indeed they could. Their database was full of names.

I began by telephoning Margaret Reichlin, an ex-seamstress who lived in Andover in Hampshire. She responded immediately by sending me one of the strangest parcels I had ever received: a thick wad of pesticides-related documents wrapped in polythene and covered in warnings written in marker-pen. 'CONTAMINATED (VICTIM'S HOME)', it read, 'BUT IN BICARB FOR MONTHS. SUGGEST YOU COPY BEFORE WORKING FROM.' She telephoned not long after to check that the parcel had arrived.

'Tell me – I'm interested. Did you feel anything?'

'Feel what?'

'Ah – I see. You're not chemically sensitized then.'

'Not so far as I know,' I replied, hiding the fact that I had no idea what she was talking about. 'I take it that you are? What symptoms should I look out for?'

'You'll know if you've got it. I get a sort of tingling in my fingertips. It's like you can . . . *feel* it in the pages.'

'Mmm,' I said, lifting one corner of the package on my desk between finger and thumb, and peering beneath it.

'It's so hard to explain to people that haven't got it,' she sighed. 'That's half the trouble. It's just so easy for the government to tell us it's all in our minds.'

As her papers exhaustively revealed, in the late 1980s Margaret Reichlin had the timbers of the cellar of her old cottage treated for woodworm. The men that came to apply the chemicals said that all she needed to do was to leave her doors open for a few hours afterwards to let any fumes disperse. But the smell of the chemicals lingered, giving her headaches and making her feel nauseous. Even her vision was affected. She moved out for a few days but it made no difference. She took the matter up with the chemicals firm. They told her she was imagining it: their products were all officially approved and safe for use around humans. So she complained to the Health and Safety Executive, but they essentially told her the same thing. Her problems didn't stop with headaches and nausea. She lost her sense of co-ordination and found she could no longer sew. She suffered from insomnia, mood swings and, eventually, mental breakdown. I was due to meet Margaret Reichlin in

Andover to discuss her experiences further, but she cancelled our meeting at the last minute, explaining that she felt too ill. The crop-spraying season had begun – a time of year, she said, when she almost always felt ill. Her initial exposure had been so extreme that her condition had become permanent; for the last eighteen years, exposure even to tiny amounts of chemicals prompted the most violent reaction. This was the true meaning of chemical sensitization.

'My life has been ruined by those chemicals,' she told me bluntly. 'I don't want compensation. All I want is for the authorities to acknowledge proper responsibility.'

I went to see another poisoning victim instead, a young woman called Georgina Downs, who lived with her parents on the edge of the village of Runcton, near Chichester. The family had built their house themselves on a 3-acre plot bought in the early 1980s, and moved in when Georgina was ten. She, too, was chemically sensitized – poisoned, she was certain, by crop-sprays absorbed or inhaled while playing in the garden as a child. Their house was surrounded by fields on three sides. She used to be a singer, but for the last five years had been campaigning full-time for a change in the law that would protect people living in rural areas from crop-spraying.

'Sorry about the stuffiness,' she said cheerfully as she welcomed me inside. 'Would you like a drink? We've got a new brand of organic water. It's lovely stuff.'

It was a hot summer's day by the time I got to Runcton. The harvest was in full swing, and all the doors and windows of the house were sealed to prevent contamination from flying chaff. She led me through the house to a snooker room at the back which served as her office. Her campaign was evidently a serious business. Every inch of the snooker table's surface was covered in orderly stacks of papers, as was her desk, all the surrounding furniture, and every surface in the snooker room's ante-room.

'If I ever do anything like this again I'll be sure to start with a proper filing system,' she sighed. 'It's too late to do anything about it now.'

Closed French windows gave on to a lawn and, immediately beyond it, a newly harvested wheat field that had been the main source of all the trouble. In the early summer of 2002 she placed a group of mannequins at the edge of the garden – a mother and children, a pregnant woman – and trained a camera on them as the field was repeatedly sprayed. She showed me the video that resulted. The field abutted the garden so closely that the boom of the crop-sprayer, still dripping with chemicals, passed virtually over the mannequins' heads. She presented the video to the Government's Advisory Committee on Pesticides. Three years on, as a direct result of her campaign, a Royal Commission on Environmental Pollution was deliberating two proposals: no-spray buffer zones around fields near people's homes, and a law obliging farmers to give residents prior notification of what, where and when they intended to spray. At present, she told me, farmers were under no legal obligation to give their neighbours any notification at all.

There wasn't much that she didn't know about agrochemical poisoning. Not long ago she and her mother had had their bodies tested for pesticide residues, and discovered that they were both packed with them. An organochlorine pesticide called Lindane scored highly: the local farmer apparently used to put it on his peas. So did several other chemicals, including organophosphates such as Diazinon, and other organochlorines including DDT.

She wasn't exaggerating when she said that her and her family's life had been blighted. As a child she frequently got blisters in her mouth, sometimes as many as twenty at a time, which were so painful that all she could eat was soup. She developed headaches, dizziness and tinnitus, and still suffered a burning sensation in her legs. When she was eighteen she was hospitalized for a month, suffering from neurological problems and acute muscle wastage. She subsequently discovered that her symptoms were typical of chemical poisoning.

Her campaign had become the family's fight. Her father Ray's eyes were burned one summer when he hurried out to close the doors of his greenhouse at the bottom of the garden: the farmer had started spraying again, and he didn't want whatever it was to spoil his prize tomatoes. He later discovered that the farmer had mixed a cocktail of three fungicides, Amistar, Opus and Corbel. He didn't venture out now when spraying was in progress without wearing gloves and an orange boiler-suit, and a filtered mask to protect his face. I laughed when Georgina showed me a photograph of him in his garden – he looked like some biological weapons specialist – but immediately wished I hadn't.

'People may take the pee out of my dad a bit, but it's no joke for him,' she said sternly.

Margaret Reichlin's bicarbonate-soaked parcel was eccentric, but I was beginning to see that the risk of agrochemical poisoning deserved to be taken seriously. Some 1.5 million people lived next to farms in Britain, Melissa's PSP-afflicted aunt Eugenie among them, and most farmland was also criss-crossed by public footpaths and rights of way. Georgina, a lone campaigner, had filled a database with the names of 750 people who had contacted her with suspected symptoms. These included everything from sore throats and eyes to eczema, asthma, allergies, myalgic encephalomyelitis (ME), Parkinson's, MS, breast cancer, leukaemia and non-Hodgkins lymphoma.

But, as Eugenie had found, the greatest difficulty faced by victims of pesticide-poisoning was proving it. Georgina explained that it was impossible to say exactly what chemical or chemicals were responsible for her own past illness because the fields around her home at Runcton had been sprayed with such a variety of compounds over the years. Her experience was typical: very few of the victims on her database were able to say with certainty that any single chemical was responsible for their complaint. This made it very difficult to achieve recognition of the problem. Officialdom required a direct causal link before it would take legislative action. Circumstantial evidence, however strong, was invariably ignored.

'The playing field is totally unlevel,' Georgina said. 'Even in murder cases in this country, people are convicted on the basis of "beyond reasonable doubt". There is plenty of reasonable doubt about the safety of agrochemicals. Yet that isn't good enough for the government's Advisory Committee on Pesticides.'

She pointed out that the precautionary principle was exercised in other parts of the world, notably in America, where seven states had established no-spray zones around schools of up to two and a half miles – although, she explained, even this distance wasn't necessarily enough because sprays could travel in the air much further than that .

'The only way really to protect the public is to ban pesticide-spraying altogether and to switch to non-chemical and natural methods,' she concluded as I got up to leave. 'Do you have children?'

'Not yet. There's one on the way, though.'

'Well, remember: developing children are the ones most at risk. Even one of the ACP lot has admitted that a foetus can be affected by amounts of agrochemicals so tiny that they are measurable in parts per trillion. No level of exposure can be considered completely safe ... Forgive me if I don't come outside to see you off.'

I wished her luck with her campaign, and she waved goodbye through the open crack of her front door as I drove away. Her demands sounded ambitious. Spray-free buffer zones of two and a half miles were all very well in America, but they would make crop-spraying almost impossible in crowded Britain. Thousands of farmers would either have to switch to non-chemical methods or go out of business. She effectively wanted to turn the clock back on half a century of agricultural technique – and I couldn't see any government agreeing to sign up to that. 'The chemist cannot be unconcerned with the many problems presented by his own action in disturbing the balance of nature,' Jack Drummond said in 1951. And yet here in West Sussex, at the beginning of the twenty-first century, the chemists appeared completely unconcerned by the possibility that their crop-sprays were not just disturbing the balance of nature, but directly harming people.

The pressure from government to maximize home production in the post-war period was hard to resist. With the nation's farmers in alliance with Whitehall, it became harder still. The voice of reason represented by the likes of Drummond might not have prevailed, even without his untimely murder in 1952. What made resistance truly futile, however, was the support for agrochemical development that came from an unexpected third party: the military.

Britain had been besieged by U-boats twice in thirty years, an experience that the generals were determined to avoid in the future. But their interest in chemicals went well beyond the strategic desirability of self-sustainability in the fields. It seems improbable now, but in 1944 it was feared that Germany might try to starve Britain by dropping Colorado beetles onto the national potato crop. After the war, the concern was that the Russians might do the same. Ample supplies of effective pesticides were therefore a matter of national self-defence.

The fear of Colorado beetles was not confined to London, or even to the West. In 1950 a pamphlet was published in Communist East Berlin blaming the US for an unseasonable plague of Colorado beetle near Zwickau. The beetles reportedly appeared a day after American planes had been seen flying over the area: 'unassailable proof', in the view of the pamphlet's author, of a 'notorious gangster diplomacy which has taken over plans for a total war of annihilation from German and Japanese fascism'. The pamphlet accused the West German chemical company IG Farben of colluding with 'Wall Street billionaires and war-mongering American imperialists'. IG Farben, it revealed, was hoping to establish a market for a new pesticide, a top-secret formulation code-named E838 that, naturally, would also be of critical military importance to the Americans, their dastardly political ringmasters. The pamphlet concluded by demanding that the UN 'take up the charges against the general staff and the government of the USA with regards to their potato beetle crimes'.

There was no evidence that anyone ever put beetle-bombing to the test. The accusation levelled by the Berlin pamphlet was typical of the paranoid spirit of the Cold War age. On the other hand, paranoia itself fuelled the drive for chemical technological supremacy. Much of the chemical experimentation of the period was therefore sponsored by the military. The 'full rein' that Attlee promised in his manifesto applied to the scientists working for the Ministry of Defence, too. The only restraint on what they could do was their imaginations – as the Lynmouth flood disaster of 1952 perhaps illustrated.

On 15 August of that year, in the middle of a heat-wave, some 90 million tons of water poured off Exmoor, Devon, creating a flash-flood that destroyed half the coastal village of Lynmouth and killed thirty-five people. News of this 'hand of God' event even pushed reports of the ten-day-old Drummond murder investigation off the front pages. A national appeal was launched to bring aid to the homeless survivors. In 2001, however, it emerged that Lynmouth had perhaps not been smitten by the hand of God after all, but by the Ministry of Defence. Declassified minutes from an air ministry meeting showed that from 5 to 15 August 1952, the RAF was engaged in a rain-making experiment called Operation Cumulus. The pilots had precipitated the rainfall by seeding clouds with various chemicals – salt, dry ice, silver iodide – which had been supplied by ICI. The minutes listed several possible military uses for the technique, including 'bogging down enemy movement', 'incrementing the water flow in rivers and streams to hinder or stop enemy crossings', and 'clearing fog from airfields'. The Lynmouth survivors called for an official enquiry into the causes of the flood, but never got one. To this day there are old people in Lynmouth who claim they saw planes circling just before the downpour.

The public of 1952 would not have believed this modern explanation for the flood, but even at this early date there were signs that the compact of trust between them and the scientists was beginning to break down. Technology – especially the new military technology that involved rockets and nuclear bombs – engendered almost as much fear and distrust as the Kremlin. 'Secret weapons', 'germ warfare' and 'Mutually Assured Destruction' were all catchphrases of the age. The preoccupation was reflected in popular culture, above all in the fashionable genre of science fiction. *The Quatermass Experiment*, a made-for-television drama broadcast live in 1953, dealt with an over-ambitious scientist and the crew of a spaceship infected by a sinister monster from another galaxy. In the 1954 hit movie *Them!* a pair of entomologists battled giant ants that had mutated after being exposed to radiation. As one of the film's heroes sagely remarked: 'When man entered the Atomic Age he opened a door to a new world. What we'll eventually find in that new world nobody can predict.' *Dr Strangelove*, the Peter Sellers film made in the 1960s but lifted from a novel written in 1958, featured a mad American general convinced that Communists had doctored the US water supply in a bid to 'sap and impurify our precious bodily fluids'. The spirit of the times may have been paranoid, but the fact that the RAF were engaged in rain-making shows that not all science fiction was fiction, and that the boffins were not necessarily as harmless as that cuddly word for them suggested.

In fact the marriage of civilian and military interests had spawned a monster with a curious characteristic. To use a sinister expression familiar from the work of United Nations weapons inspectors in Iraq in the late 1990s, the new agrochemicals were 'dual use'. Herbicides could be used by farmers to keep weeds at bay, thus maximizing crop production to help feed the nation; but they could also be used offensively, to destroy the enemy's crops, or as a defoliant to spoil their cover, *à la* Agent Orange. Pesticides were the same: they could be used by farmers and gardeners to maximize food production, but also by armies in jungles to fend off mosquitoes.

In one instance, a pesticide was even a tool of genocide: the cyanide-based formulation Zyklon-B, the development history of which neatly illustrates the Janus-faced nature of agrochemicals. Invented as an insecticide in the 1920s by the Nobel Prize-winning chemist Fritz Haber,

Zyklon-B was originally deployed at Auschwitz for delousing inmates in order to control typhus. In 1941, of course, the Nazis found a rather different use for it. At least half a million Jews were killed by Zyklon-B in the Auschwitz gas chambers alone. Haber, ironically, was himself a Jew who had been forced to flee Hitler's regime in 1933, despite his earlier voluntary conversion from Judaism. Among those killed at Auschwitz were several members of Haber's own family.

Haber's life was emblematic in other ways of the sometimes cataclysmic consequences of the marriage of scientific and military interests. On 22 April 1915, at Ypres, he had personally overseen the first poison gas attack in modern military history. The gas used was chlorine: 168 tons of his special preparation were released over a 4-mile front, killing some 350, mainly French, troops within ten minutes and maiming 7000 others. Back in Berlin, Haber was the hero of the hour – although not to his wife Clara, who was so appalled by what her husband had done that, at a dinner party thrown in his honour, she shot herself dead with his service revolver. The following day Haber, evidently the toughest kind of patriot, left Berlin for the Eastern Front to oversee further gas attacks against the Russians. The inventor of the first true Weapon of Mass Destruction died in Basle in 1934.

In the future, the dual nature of agrochemicals meant that they could be developed for the military – or, indeed, clandestinely exported – under cover of some purported civilian application, as dictators like Saddam Hussein were quick to realize. In the 1950s it would have been hard even for a willing government to regulate an industry that sometimes worked for agriculture, sometimes for the military, or (in the case of ICI) for both at the same time. The defence of the realm during the Cold War was necessarily a covert business. As I was to discover, the secrecy that surrounded the development of agrochemicals had much to do with the mysterious death of Drummond and his family; it was also more responsible than I'd ever suspected for the chemical contamination of mine.

Chapter 4

Amelia's Chemical World

'Wherefore let us neither with the impudent call diet a frivolous
knowledge, or a curious science with the imprudent: but embrace it
as the leader to perfit health, (which as the wise man saith) is above
gold, and a sound body above all riches.'

Thomas Muffet (1655), quoted in *The Englishman's Food*

Our daughter Amelia was born in the spring of 2005. She wasn't too big
or too small, she had all the right number of digits and limbs, and
everyone agreed with us that she was beautiful. But that didn't stop us
from worrying about the chemical world we had brought her into. In fact,
from the moment we first carried her out of the hospital, a hundred-yard
dash along a road choked with rush-hour traffic, we both felt a deep-
seated urge to shield her. It felt intrinsically wrong to be exposing
something so young, so vulnerable and so patently uncontaminated to
the noise and pollution of bus engines. Of course we could not expect to
preserve our baby's shiny newness for ever. But did the downhill slide
into the mucky swamp of the world have to begin quite so soon? Neither
of us voiced this neurosis, yet I could tell from Melissa's face as she
carried our baby to the car that the perfect happiness I wanted her to feel
was compromised by it.

This was partly my fault. I had discovered a lot about chemical
contamination during the months of Melissa's pregnancy, and I hadn't
exactly spared her the grisly details. As modern Westerners it seemed

beyond doubt that we were tainted with toxins. Much more disturbing was my discovery in a book called *Pandora's Poison*, a closely argued attack on the international chlorine industry by a biologist called Joe Thornton, that Melissa's 'chemical load' would almost certainly be passed on to Amelia via her breast milk.

This applied especially to the organochlorine pesticides which, as Thornton explained, were generally soluble in human body fat, and tended to 'bio-accumulate' there. The consequences for the accumulator's health – cancer, endocrine disruption, reproductive problems – were potentially calamitous. The body did get rid of organochlorine contaminants naturally, but only very slowly over the course of many years, or even a lifetime. Expressing milk, it appeared, was one of the few ways that the body was able to flush them out faster. Research suggested that a first-born, breast-fed child could expect to inherit up to 30 per cent of the chemical load of its mother, decreasing to 20 per cent for the second born, and to 15 per cent for the third.

No-one could yet say what the long-term effects of such an inheritance might be. The phenomenon was still too new. Nevertheless, the organochlorines found in the tissues and fluids of the North American population as a whole were so numerous that Thornton listed them as an appendix that continued for six and half pages. The contamination of the Arctic Inuits was a particular *cause célèbre*. Scientists had discovered that the typical Inuit infant's intake of some organochlorines via breast milk was forty-eight times the Canadian government's 'tolerable daily intake' for adults. The reason was the pollution of seal-meat, an Inuit staple with a particularly high fat content. As a consequence, the Inuit tradition of breast-feeding babies for up to a year had been forced to a hasty end.

Melissa had been determined to breast-feed rather than, as she put it, 'stuff her baby full of nasty artificial formula'. The news that her breast milk might be chlorinated filled her with paranoid gloom.

'And to think I thought I wouldn't have to worry about what I was feeding her for at least the first six months,' she groaned.

Yet in the end she decided not to switch to formula, and I did not argue. The state-employed health visitors who kept an eye on Melissa in the first days after the birth were universal in their belief that breast-feeding was best. Mother's milk, they insisted, contained antibodies and a finely tuned balance of essential nutrients that no formula could hope to recreate. We allowed ourselves to be swayed by their arguments, and Melissa carried on as before. She even persevered through three attacks of mastitis. Breast-feeding, I understood, was something that she badly wanted – and her maternal instinct commanded respect.

The issue still niggled me, though. The vehemence with which some of the maternity nurses made the case for breast-feeding jarred. They were kindly, uncomplicated and dedicated young women, mostly, yet I couldn't shake the feeling that they had somehow been indoctrinated. The more fervent ones annoyed Melissa, who called them 'breast Nazis', and I knew what she meant. One of them dealt only in comfortable dogma and resisted all debate, particularly (or so it seemed to me) when this was offered by me, the mere father.

'Research has shown that breast-fed babies are less likely to become overweight or obese and have a lower risk of developing heart disease in later life,' she said, skewering me with a disapproving eye. 'I promise you: breast is best.'

This was the policy of the World Health Organization, word for word. The WHO's authority was so indisputable that the formula manufacturers like SMA, Hipp and Milupa Aptamil were obliged to print the breast-is-best incantation on their tins – perhaps the only industry in the world that advertised its principal rival on its own packaging. Yet if breast milk was contaminated it didn't deserve such superlative description. 'Breast is probably better' would have been a more honest slogan, or 'Breast may be the lesser of two evils'. Melissa and I were intelligent parents who could decide for ourselves. What right did the WHO have to dictate to us? Clarity, of course, was essential when setting a global policy. Disseminating the ambiguous truth would not be helpful in the overstretched mud-hut maternity clinics of East Africa. But here in the West, the breezy confidence that the WHO placed in breast-feeding felt patronizing, arrogant and misplaced. It seemed a great tragedy that mother's milk, the original staff of life, had become yet another source of fear. The troubling reality was that at the beginning of the twenty-first century our daughter had effectively been born into a chemical food scare.

I wondered for weeks what organochlorines might have bio-accumulated in the fatty tissues of Melissa's body over the years, and indeed in mine. There was only one way to find out: we would have to get ourselves tested, just as Georgina Downs had done. I rang her, got the number of a specialist medical unit called Biolab, and was soon talking to the director of the unit, a Dr John McLaren-Howard DSc.

'We're seeing a rising number of patients who appear to have pesticide-related problems,' he said. 'A screening costs £75. It's a simple procedure – just a quick jab in the backside to extract a fat sample. You'll have to get your GP to refer you, though. General Medical Council rules, I'm afraid.'

I explained that my wife was breast-feeding and asked if we could get her milk tested too. He said he couldn't see why not.

'Let me get this straight,' said Melissa when I put it to her. 'I've been a mother for exactly a month, and you want me to do *what*?'

'A pesticides test. It won't take long. Consider it an exercise in reassurance.'

'Reassurance? You call having some . . . some *quack* stick a needle in my bum reassuring?'

'It's in the interests of science,' I said. 'And when it's over you'll know your breast milk is nice and pure for Amelia.'

'Oh God, my breast milk as well. Do I have to?'

'Of course not. But if you don't you'll never be sure, will you?'

'I hate needles.'

'Oh go on, please? It might be fun.'

She looked at me with one eyebrow raised, and said nothing.

'I'll do it purely out of love,' she said finally, 'so long as you buy me dinner afterwards.'

Persuading our doctors to refer us to Biolab proved easier said than done. Melissa and I had different GPs, and neither of them had heard of Biolab or ever been asked to refer a patient for a pesticides test. My GP was fascinated and agreed to help at once, but Melissa's would have nothing to do with it, even after thinking about it for a week.

'We wouldn't have a clue how to analyse the results,' she said. 'I really don't feel comfortable with it.'

I tried to convince her that she was obstructing a ground-breaking piece of medical research, but it did no good.

'Everyone has their comfort levels,' she said primly.

In the end we had to resort to a friendly health visitor, who was happy to sign once I explained that we would also be screening Melissa's breast milk.

We found Biolab at the eastern end of Weymouth Street in London W1, on the outermost fringes of the district of medical respectability around Harley Street. Dr McLaren-Howard's qualification was from the American College of Nutrition, an institution I had never heard of, but any misgivings were allayed when I met him. He was clearly no quack. He remembered Georgina Downs, and had followed the recent debate on crop-sprays closely in the press. Indeed, Biolab had submitted information to the Royal Commission on Environmental Protection and expected to do so again in the near future.

'It's hard to say how bad a given organochlorine is for a person,' he told me. 'No-one really knows, because different molecular structures will bind with different organochlorines in different ways. Toxicity depends on an individual's DNA.'

From the scientific point of view, all that one could say for sure about organochlorines was that they were 'likely' contributors to a potential cocktail effect in the human body. Establishing the extent of their contribution would probably never be possible.

'Cocktail effect theory is still not taken very seriously, which I find worrying. I'm old enough to remember the fight to get PCB flame-retardants banned in the 1970s. But PCBs have been replaced by PBBs, which merely swap bromide for the chlorine element and cause exactly the same problems. We see a lot of PBB contamination here at Biolab. I can understand why industry would want to find a way around a ban: that's what commercial enterprises do. But I can't understand why the government supports them. PBBs are incorporated *by law* in the flame-retardants used in the furniture that we sit and lie around in all day . . . That's what really gives me the collywobbles.'

After a long wait we were led into a consulting room where we were seen to by a bespectacled nurse from Austria.

'Pesticides test? *Sehr gut*,' she said, pulling on a surgical glove with a resounding snap.

'It's not a big needle, is it?' said Melissa nervously.

'No, no. We only need a very small sample.'

I grinned fixedly at Melissa as, seconds later, the nurse slid a needle into the subcutaneous fat in my buttock. Melissa looked glum when her turn came, and glummer still as she handed over a sealed pot of newly-expressed breast milk.

'You live in London?' said the nurse. '*Ach*! I think you will be all right. London is safer to live in than the countryside these days. There are so many pesticides in the countryside.'

She wasn't wrong. According to Michael Meacher, the area of crops sprayed with pesticides in the UK had increased by a million hectares since the mid-1990s. Neither Melissa nor I had lived in the countryside in the last ten years, which was comforting. On the other hand, we had both gone on umpteen country holidays in our lifetimes, and had both attended rural boarding schools as children; and because organochlorines took so long to break down in the human body, we were looking for evidence of contamination that could have taken place as long ago as the late 1960s or early 1970s. Back out on the pavement I gave Melissa a kiss on the cheek.

'That wasn't so bad, was it?' I said. 'You've struck a great blow for science. A classic piece of self-experimentation! Jack Drummond would be proud of you. *I'm* proud of you.'

'Thank you,' she said, 'but don't think for one minute that that is an acceptable substitute for buying me dinner.'

The test results came through a few days later. I honestly didn't expect them to reveal anything dramatic. There would be traces of pesticides no doubt, but not much more than that, for we were both sure that we had never been exposed to as many crop-sprays as Georgina Downs. All the same, I found myself tearing open my envelope as impatiently as a schoolboy who had just been posted his exam results.

It took a few seconds to understand what I was looking at. Each tested chemical had been given a 'Provisional Limit of Acceptability' – a reminder of science's inability to establish precisely how much of a given chemical was bad for you, just as John McLaren-Howard had said. On the other hand, the provisional limit in each case was the highest figure from a control range of fifty-seven separate medical studies, which lent it a certain credibility. The upper limit for Lindane was 0.05 mg per kg of fat. My fat, I was horrified to see, contained three times that figure: 0.15 mg. This was far less than Georgina Downs, whose test had revealed 0.4 mg per kg, but I wasn't comforted. Alone among the test list of chemicals, Lindane carried a footnote that read: 'may be hazardous at ANY level'. My interest in pesticides-poisoning had just turned unpleasantly personal.

It didn't stop there. My listing for Pentachlorophenol, a fungicide once widely used as a wood preservative (but banned after it was linked to liver and kidney damage), was 50 per cent over the limit of acceptability. As for 'PBB (BDE) flame-retardants', I could hardly bear to look: 0.22 mg per kg, against a limit of acceptability of 0.05 mg. I also contained significantly high levels of DDT, DDE, HCB, PCBs, p-Dichlorobenzene, Dieldrin and Chlordane. The fact that I only contained a 'trace' of Mirex and DDD was not consoling. The test was a confirmation of all the scary statistics: I was a walking laboratory crucible.

Melissa's results arrived after mine. There was another flurry of envelope-opening. It appeared that she, too, contained too many flame-retardants: 0.14 mg per kg compared to the limit of 0.05. Yet overall her body was inexplicably purer than mine. There were traces of most of the same chemicals, including Lindane, although the levels were less in each case. A second page was dedicated to Melissa's breast milk. All the same chemicals were present. As expected the levels here were lower still, but it was still the most depressing page to read. Our newborn baby's diet contained DDT, DDD, DDE, HCB, PCBs, PBB (BDE) flame-retardants, p-Dichlorobenzene, Carbaryl, Chlordane and, of course, Lindane. It was astounding to realize that the use of some of these chemicals, DDT among them, had been banned in Britain for at least twenty years. John McLaren-Howard had scrawled a note at the bottom of the breast milk report that did nothing to cheer Melissa up. 'Results are well within background exposure levels,' it read.

'Oh God,' said Melissa, hiding her face in her hands. 'I think I've just killed our baby.'

I had a hunch that it was going to take more than dinner in a restaurant to restore her equanimity.

The contaminant that bothered me most was my triple-limit dose of Lindane. Until I met Georgina Downs I had never heard of this substance. I knew it was an organochlorine pesticide like DDT, but still had no real understanding of what that meant, nor any idea of how so much of it had found its way into my body. Thanks to the sinister note at the bottom of the Biolab report, however, I was more than a little anxious to find out.

There was plenty of information available online. Lindane, I learned, was one of the earliest organochlorines, developed like DDT during World War Two. Named after the Dutch chemist Teunis van der Linden, who discovered it in 1912, it was an odourless white crystal, cheap to manufacture and up to twenty times more lethal to insects than DDT. It was also potentially more toxic to humans than DDT. It was used for almost half a century in the UK for the control of insects in cereal crops, grassland, potatoes, stored grain, fruit and forestry. According to government figures it was still one of the seven most widely used pesticides in Britain in 1989. It was also used to treat woodworm and, until the mid-1990s, to kill lice on the heads of children, particularly in America.

Its persistence in the environment had led to its designation as one of the 'Dirty Dozen' chemicals known as Persistent Organic Pollutants, or POPs, that had been singled out for global elimination by the United Nations in 1996. After a sustained campaign by environmentalists and health groups as well as pressure from the European Union, Britain finally placed severe restrictions on its use in 1999. It was nasty stuff all right. The only debate among scientists was how much of it was harmful to human health. Decades of research had shown that it was linked to a host of serious health problems: neurological disorders, liver and kidney damage, leukaemia, aplastic anaemia – and brain cancer in children using Lindane shampoo. The strongest link was to breast cancer, a particular problem in Britain, where cases have risen by 80 per cent in the last thirty years – one of the highest rates in the world. In parts of Lincolnshire, where it was once used extensively on sugar beet to kill European crane fly, the incidence of breast cancer in 1995 was found to be 40 per cent higher than the already high national average.

'That's all very interesting,' said Melissa, breast-feeding the baby, 'but what I want really to know is: how do I get rid of it?'

'Apart from expressing it in your milk, you mean?'

'I don't think that's funny.'

I rang John McLaren-Howard again for advice.

'Infrared sauna is supposed to be quite effective,' he said cheerfully. 'It mimics the energy emitted naturally by the body, so the heat gets deeper into your fat cells than a conventional sauna, and the toxins are sweated out on the skin. You have to scrub yourself in the shower afterwards though, otherwise the toxins are reabsorbed.'

'I see . . . so is it worth the trouble? What I mean to say is, how worried should we be about Lindane in our bodies?'

'Impossible to say. Obviously you'd be better off without it. But as I said before, toxicity would depend on your individual DNA.'

'And where does one go for an infrared sauna in London?'

'I'm afraid I've no idea.'

I relayed the news to Melissa, who again hid her face in her hands.

'What the hell is an infrared sauna? It sounds like some kind of microwave.'

'Could be. I'll let you know when I've found one. *If* I find one.'

'So now we've got to cook ourselves until we pop, like popcorn. God, I wish you'd never started this chemicals business.'

'Ignorance was bliss, wasn't it? On the other hand, I haven't been in a sauna for years. It might be a laugh.'

'I bet this infrared thingy isn't recommended for breast-feeding mothers. It'll probably make my milk boil.'

'Oh, come on. We could speak in absurd Swedish accents and flog each other's naked bodies with birch twigs.'

'You wish,' she muttered.

Working out how to detoxify our bodies could wait. Privately, I was just as interested in discovering how Lindane had got into our bodies in the first place. Lindane contamination was not unusual. Indeed, John McLaren-Howard had said that he had seen rising levels of it among the members of the public that Biolab had tested. Lindane had a 'half-life' in the human body of about fifteen years, which meant that I could have been exposed to it at any time in the thirty-eight years of my life.

'Who knows?' McLaren-Howard said when I asked him to suggest a source. 'Your level is high, but not that high. I've seen people with direct and recent exposure who have ten times as much in their fat cells. You could have got it from wading through a recently sprayed cornfield, or from eating just one heavily sprayed vegetable ages ago.'

Or, it now occurred to me, from eating farmed Scottish salmon. I hadn't forgotten about the scare the previous year, and the claim by Professor Ronald Hites of Indiana University that farmed Scottish salmon contained higher levels of fourteen banned agrochemicals than anywhere else in the world. I downloaded the Hites report from the Internet for a closer look, and immediately struck gold: Lindane was on the list. So, for that matter, were four other substances that had shown up in my Biolab test: DDT, Dieldrin, Chlordane and Mirex. All fourteen of the banned agrochemicals, I now noticed, were also organochlorines.

As I understood it, Scotland's salmon farmers routinely fed their stock with Canthaxanthin, the dye that had been linked to eye problems in children. That seemed cynical enough. Could they really be such monsters as to employ all these other dangerous chemicals as well? And if so, how and why were they allowed to get away with it?

I went to Scotland to try to find out. An ex-salmon farmer called Johnny Parry, whose sister was married to my uncle, agreed to put me up and explain how salmon farming worked. He was the right man for it. In 2000 Johnny had been accused of using a pesticide for which he had no licence. After nearly twenty years as a salmon farmer he had effectively been driven out of business, although he was still a member of the Wester Ross Fisheries Trust.

'The danger of chemical poisoning is grossly overdone,' he told me. 'Of course there are chemicals in salmon. You couldn't farm without them. But that's true of all intensive animal husbandry. Salmon farming is neither better nor worse than any other kind of farming.'

'But what about Canthaxanthin? Did you know it was linked to eye problems in children?'

He shook his head impatiently. 'Canthaxanthin isn't around any more. These days they use Astaxanthin. Anyway, you'd have to eat impossible amounts of it before there was any health risk.'

He was equally dismissive of the Cassandra from Indiana. None of the organochlorines that the Americans had tested for, he insisted, had ever been used on his or any other fish farm that he knew of.

'Are you sure that report was objective?' he added. 'I bet it was funded by an ecologist group in Canada or somewhere.'

We were standing on a steep, heathery promontory called Stattic Point, at the western tip of Little Loch Broom just south of Ullapool. It was drizzling in the proper Scots way. Water dripped from the end of Johnny's untamed beard, although the rain was less troublesome than the midges, which rose up from the heather in clouds. The view was staggering, even on this murky day. Five miles away, the Summer Isles cracked the horizon. Beyond that was the open Atlantic; there was no other land mass between here and Iceland, 500 miles away at least to the north-east. But it was the foreground that had drawn us to this numinous place. In the sea-loch far below us a dozen vast circular cages, each 50 metres across, were arranged in two parallel lines of six. To one side floated a windowless control room that was painted a forbidding battleship grey. With the incoming tide breaking around its prow, its ellipsoidal shape looked a lot like the conning tower of a surfacing submarine.

This, Johnny wanted me to know, was the reality of modern salmon farming. Some 65 million fish a year were produced in Scotland in this way – just a small contribution to a global market that was worth more than $4bn. A nautically minded cousin of mine once called salmon 'sea-chicken'. Now I could see why, for the operation below us was undoubtedly the marine equivalent of a battery farm. Like almost every Scottish salmon farm, it was run by the Dutch-owned company Marine Harvest, the world's largest fish-farm operator. A quarter of this company, revealingly enough, was owned by Stolt-Nielsen SA, who were not fishmongers or farmers or even food-retailers, but specialists in the transportation of liquid chemicals.

The salmon, Johnny said, were all fed by computer now. Small independent operators like him were a thing of the past. When he went into the business in the 1980s he did so alone, with a single cage held together with rope and wood, and fed his fish from sacks tipped in from the side of a pitching dinghy. Marine Harvest, by contrast, ran fish farms in eight countries on five continents and sold €850m of salmon and other farmed fish a year. The speed with which salmon farming had been industrialized was awe-inspiring. Even with computerization they managed to employ 6000 people.

'You'd never be able to set up on your own these days. They wouldn't let you. The Scottish salmon industry is the most regulated in the world ... Farmers have to meet forty-eight separate regulatory requirements. You wouldn't believe the paperwork.'

Johnny was evidently not the type to be bound by regulations. It was the wildness of the Highlands that had drawn him, an Englishman, to this remote corner of Scotland in the first place. It was clear that industrialization had taken all the fun out of salmon farming since then. His run-in with the authorities in Edinburgh began when he was reported by an employee, Jackie McKenzie, whom he had ordered to slip an insecticide into the salmon cages in order to kill sea-lice, the carnivorous parasite that is the bane of all salmon farmers. The insecticide was based on a synthetic pyrethroid, Cypermethrin, the use of which required a licence that Johnny had not been granted. Cypermethrin was not only highly toxic to sea-life: it was another possible carcinogen and suspected hormone disruptor in humans.

He described what happened next as a 'witch-hunt'. The anti-salmon-farm lobby had long suspected the farmers of environmental malpractice, which they partly blamed for the catastrophic collapse in wild salmon stocks on the west coast in recent years, and this was the first hard evidence of it. For reasons of ancient history the well-being of salmon was an emotive issue in Scotland. The fish was a symbol of magic and wisdom in Celtic mythology. The Salmon Farm Protest Group, led by Bruce Sandison, the former angling correspondent of the *Scotsman*, appealed directly to Scotland's sense of its misty Pictish past on the masthead of its website which read: 'An rud bhios na do bhroin, cha bhi e na do thiomhnadh – That which you have wasted will not be there for future generations'. There were wags in Edinburgh who surmised that the leader of the Scottish National Party, Alex Salmond, owed much of his success to his surname. It was hardly surprising that English Johnny was pilloried in the Scottish press.

Five years on, the swirl of emotion generated by the episode had still not faded. Jackie McKenzie, a Hepatitis C sufferer, blamed Cypermethrin contamination for his continuing ill-health and was still pursuing the matter through the courts. He accused his former boss of greed and exploitation, but after meeting Johnny and his family I knew this wasn't true. Johnny was a free spirit, a charming and vigorous entrepreneur who had tried as best he could to make a living from the sea. He was no evil exploiter. His style was merely a little cavalier. According to Jackie McKenzie, he used to handle chemicals with gloves full of holes, and opened bottles of Cypermethrin with his teeth.

His attitude towards health and safety regulations aside, Johnny's crime was not that he had used Cypermethrin, but that he had used it without a licence. More than 300 Cypermethrin licences were issued by SEPA, the Scottish Environmental Protection Agency, between 1998 and 2004. The use of chemicals by salmon farmers enjoyed the same official endorsement that the consumption of their product did by the FSA in London. It was easy to understand why Johnny might have felt inclined to deceive the SEPA bureaucrats. He had a living to make, and his valuable stock was being eaten alive by parasites.

The view changed as I stumbled on behind him through the soaking heather of Stattic Point, revealing a mile-long island close to the western shore. This was Gruinard, a place infamous in the annals of biological warfare. In 1942 the Ministry of Defence chose it as a suitable site for an experimental release of anthrax, a deadly bacterium that quickly wiped out a flock of sheep.

'Our family were the first to picnic there when it was reopened,' said Johnny proudly. 'Anthrax is nothing to worry about. It's a cattle spore that occurs all the time in nature.'

I was impressed by his insouciance. I later read that, according to the US National Academy of Sciences, a kilo of anthrax released over a city the size of, say, Paris could kill over 120,000 people. The contaminated island was not judged safe for humans until 1990, when a junior defence minister made the half-mile journey from the mainland to remove the MoD's red warning sign. It was another illustration of the link between the 1940s and the present day. Nowhere in Britain, it seemed, was free of the industrial legacy of war – not even a place as remote as Wester Ross.

None of this, however, explained the presence of Lindane in farmed Scottish salmon. Johnny Parry was categorical: it had never been used in the fight against sea-lice or any other pest or parasite that afflicted the fish. Indeed, he had only vaguely heard of Lindane, and was amazed to hear about its bio-accumulation in my body. I found my answer eventually in the place I should have looked first – in Joe Thornton's book on the international chlorine industry, *Pandora's Poison*.

In common with other organochlorine pesticides, Lindane was only slightly water-soluble and never broke down easily in the environment. Instead it tended to travel and spread when it was released. When applied to field crops a high proportion of it – up to 90 per cent, according to some studies – entered the atmosphere and was later deposited by rain. Lindane also leached directly into ground water, or entered rivers and oceans as surface run-off. After half a century, therefore, Lindane had spread literally everywhere. In 1995 scientists analysed tree-bark from ninety sites around the world and found Lindane present at all of them. The concentrations were naturally highest in those industrialized nations where use had been heaviest, but it was also found in some of the world's most remote regions – the rainforests of Ecuador, the savannas of Togo, Guam, Tasmania and the Marshall Islands.

Environmental pollution had never much interested me before. It had been a fashionable issue to worry about in my student years, but I tended not to be among the hand-wringers when an oil tanker spilled its load or a new hole was discovered in the ozone layer. Now I plunged in with the eagerness of a man making up lost time.

'So you've become an eco-warrior,' said Melissa, back in London. 'I never thought going to Scotland for a couple of days could have such an effect.'

'I'm not about to handcuff myself to a tree. I just want to know if it's OK to eat salmon or not. Don't you want to know what you're putting in your mouth?'

'I confess there are times when I'd almost rather not,' she sighed.

Once in the sea, Lindane tended to float around until it got eaten, bio-accumulating – and bio-concentrating – in the fatty tissues of living organisms as it moved up the food chain. A study in the North Pacific found that zooplankton carried organochlorine concentrations 6400 times greater than in the water in which they were swimming. Lantern-fish, which ate zooplankton, carried concentrations 170,000 greater. For squid, which ate lantern-fish, the figure was 240,000. But for striped dolphin, the unfortunate beasts that ate squid, the bio-concentration factor was a staggering 13 to 37 million times greater.

Salmon lived near the top of their food chain so it followed that Lindane was bio-concentrating alarmingly in their fat cells, too. In Scotland, I had learned, farmed salmon were typically fed on fish meal made of ground-up sand eels from the North Sea. In 1985 an International Conference on the Protection of the North Sea agreed to reduce emissions of a number of toxic chemicals, including Lindane, by 50 per cent over the following ten years. The UK failed spectacularly to meet its target. In fact in a single year, between 1990 and 1991, emissions of Lindane into the North Sea from the UK *increased* by 50 per cent. Here at last was an explanation for the high levels of Lindane found in farmed salmon.

The proof, if one cared to look for it, was in the Hites study. For the sake of comparison, Hites had tested wild salmon for contaminants, too

– and found just as many organochlorines in their bodies. On average, admittedly, the levels of these organochlorines were about one-tenth of those found in farmed salmon, for the simple reason that the diet of wild fish is usually more varied – but not always. In one case, indeed, the level of Lindane found in a wild salmon's fat cells was actually higher than in some farmed fish. None of this was reported by the press at the time of the food scare. But the fact remained that the contamination of the King of Fish was not really the fault of the farmers. Thanks to man's pollution of the planet, even salmon left to their own devices were contaminated, and no salmon was truly clean. According to the Hites report, the least contaminated salmon in the world was the wild Alaskan variety, which in Britain generally came in cans. Melissa did not take this news well.

'Bloody hell,' she said. 'I hate tinned food. I'm not sure I've even got an opener.'

'I reckon it's OK to eat non-tinned salmon. It's just that you shouldn't eat it too often, that's all. And definitely not the farmed stuff. It's important to keep a sense of proportion, remember?'

'But if you want to eat oily fish, there are plenty of other species from lower down the food chain that are cleaner, right? Herring and mackerel, for instance. Or sprats.'

'Sprats? Have you ever actually eaten sprats?'

'No. Have you?'

'Definitely not. But I do know a nursery rhyme. "Jack Sprat could eat no . . ."'

'Oh, stop!'

I suspected that teriyaki salmon in a wasabi mash would not be reappearing on our kitchen table any time soon.

What was the root cause of the cellular ruination of the world's salmon? The answer, yet again, was the failure of agrochemists in the 1940s adequately to investigate the potential side-effects of their new products. It was the British – specifically, ICI – who first developed

Lindane into a useable insecticide. Lindane was a molecular variant, or isomer, of benzene hexachloride, also known as hexachlorocyclohexane or HCH, which itself had been discovered by Michael Faraday, the genius from Newington Butts who invented the dynamo, the transformer and the direct current motor. In 1825 Faraday bubbled chlorine through benzene in sunlight, resulting in what he described as a 'tenacious triple compound of chlorine, carbon and hydrogen'.

HCH was a mixture of several isomers and other complex chlorinated structures, but only the 'gamma' isomer, which could be separated from the mixture by the use of solvents, was shown to have true insecticidal properties. In the best boffin tradition the usefulness of gamma-HCH was discovered almost by accident. In 1942, ICI launched a programme at their agricultural research station at Jealott's Hill, Berkshire, to find a new moth repellent. Since the early nineteenth century the standard remedy for moth had been derris powder, a root extract from the tropics, but imports had come to a halt following the Japanese occupation of Malaya. A large batch of HCH happened to be available. According to one corporate history, ICI's research staff tended to look on pesticide tests as a 'suitable destination for any intractable and evil-smelling residue for which no other use could be envisaged'. The HCH was duly sent along to the testing room, where one Saturday morning it was sprinkled on the floor next to a cage full of locusts. By Monday, all the locusts were dead. HCH was soon being tested in various forms and found to be lethal to all sorts of insects – raspberry beetles, flea beetles on cabbages, aphids on hops, and wireworm in cereals and potatoes.

It was some time before the researchers realized that the true toxicity of HCH lay only in its gamma isomer. HCH was originally dubbed '666', a Satanic-sounding codename that might have been designed to excite latter-day conspiracy theorists, but in reality was a prosaic truncation of HCH's chemical formula, $C_6H_6Cl_6$. As awareness grew of the role of the gamma isomer, 666 was renamed 'Gammexane'. The only problem with the new product – or so it seemed then – was that it tended to make food taste 'musty'. (This was probably due to imperfections in the extraction process. The pure gamma-isomer is practically tasteless: subsequent tests showed mustiness to be a characteristic of unseparated or 'technical' HCH.) Twice a day a bell rang at Jealott's Hill, and white-coated researchers would gather at the 'taint kitchen'. Here they would munch dutifully through carefully numbered platefuls of mashed potato, swede, carrots, onions, beets, fruit, chicken and eggs. They even tested chips fried in fat taken from chickens fed on Gammexane-treated grain. The flavour of potatoes was said to be particularly badly affected.

One wonders if those researchers would have been quite so amateurish if they had known what the world now does about Lindane. There is no evidence that ICI ever tested their new product for any side-effect other than taste. It was the very opposite of the 'wide range of tests' called for by Jack Drummond. The haste with which the new product was brought to market was due, once again, to the war. There were two reasons, the first military. Lindane was very effective against mosquitoes – significantly more effective, in fact, than DDT. Lindane might easily have become the household name that DDT once was. In the end, ICI's timing was just unlucky. The British army had begun jungle trials of DDT before ICI could draw attention to their own product. After the war, the WHO studied Lindane's effectiveness against mosquitoes, but by then attention had shifted to other types of insecticide.

The second reason was domestic. The speedy development of anything that might help Britain to Dig for Victory was a matter of national survival – and Lindane was a magic bullet against weevil and wireworm, the enemies of wheat and potatoes that were the most important home crops of all. What did it matter if it made potatoes taste nasty? Quantity of crop production was what mattered now, not quality. Short-cuts were encouraged; the famous catchphrase of the 1940s, 'Don't you know there's a war on?', covered a multitude of sins.

The use of Lindane was widespread by 1946 both at home and abroad. The speed with which ICI's formula was picked up and copied by foreign rivals was another function of the war. The government suspected from the outset that it might have important military uses, just as they had with ICI's other ground-breaking discovery of the period, the selective hormone weed-killer MCPA – and so banned the company from the normal filing of patents overseas.

As before, the precaution was futile. The Jealott's Hill team didn't know it in 1942, but French and American scientists coincidentally had also noticed the insecticidal properties of the gamma isomer of HCH and conducted their own experiments. They were able to combine their research with ICI's and to come up with their own versions of Gammexane. From a commercial point of view, therefore, the unpatented product was never a great success for ICI, and their brand name for the new product didn't stick. By the 1990s the International Agency for Research on Cancer listed eighty-nine brand synonyms for the gamma isomer of HCH, although it was always more commonly known by its original name, Lindane.

࿔ ࿔

Synonyms for Lindane

Aalindan

Aficide

Agrocide

Agrocide III

Agrocide WP

Ameisenmittel Merck

Ameisentod

Aparasin

Aphtiria

Aplidal

Arbitex

BBH

Ben-Hex

Bentox 10

γ-Benzene hexachloride

γ-BHC

Bexol

Celanex

Chloresene

Codechine

DBH

Detmol-extrakt

Devoran

Dol granule

Drill tox-spezial aglukon

ENT 7796

Entomoxan

Forlin

Gamacid

Gamaphex

Gammalin

Gammalin 20

Gammaterr

Gammexane

Gexane

HCH

γ-HCH

Heclotox

Hexa

Hexachloran

Hexachloran-gamma

Hexachlorane

Hexachlorane-gamma

γ-Hexachlorobenzene

γ-Hexachlorocyclohexane

γ-1,2,3,4,5,6-Hexachlorocyclohexane

Hexatox

Hexaverm

Hexicide

Hexyclan

HGI

Hortex

Isotox

Jacutin

Kokotine

Kwell

Lendine

Lentox

Lidenal

Lindafor

Lindagam

γ-Lindane

Lindatox

Lindosep

Lintox

Lorexane

Milbol 49

Mszycol

Neo-scabicidol

Nexen FB

Nexit

Nexit-stark

Nexol-E

Nicochloran

Novigam

Omnitox

Ovadziak

Owadziak

Pedraczak

Pflanzol

Quellada

Sang-gamma

Silvanol

Sprehpflanzol

Spritz-Rapidin

Streunex

TAP 85

Tri-6

Viton

৵ ৵

For two months after my visit to Scotland, I was convinced that salmon or some other item in my past diet was responsible for the triple-limit Lindane in my body. A vegetable, a fruit, a fish, a ready-meal – who knew? There didn't seem much point in worrying about a mistake or an accident that belonged to my bachelor past. What mattered was that my diet, and indeed my whole lifestyle, had changed dramatically since Amelia's birth. The contamination would not be repeated. I had never felt fitter. I decided to run the London Marathon for charity and bought a pair of running shoes from a shop called *Run and Become*. Training for this event required a degree of dietary self-discipline – and nutritional self-education – of which Drummond would have approved. On my longer training runs I carried along the refreshments recommended by *Run and Become* – densely packed 'power-bars' and hi-glucose drinks in sachets – and was regularly astounded by the speed with which they restored my tired body. The old saying 'You are what you eat' was revealed to be truer than I had ever suspected. Melissa came to support me on the big day, popping out of the crowd at the 23-mile mark with Amelia gurgling in a sling on her chest. It was a moment of the purest vindication for my happy new life.

I was wrong about the primary source of my Lindane contamination, though. Not long after the marathon, a chance conversation with an uncle, Jeremy Hughes, set me on a new track. Jeremy was the brother-in-law of Johnny Parry, the ex-salmon farmer in Wester Ross. Until 1977 he had farmed 400 acres of wheat and barley at Furneaux Pelham in Hertfordshire, before handing over to his older brother Kit. Both brothers harvested in the same way. The grain was brought to a drier, a high silver silo with a hot air cushion at the bottom, which tumbled it until all the moisture evaporated.

'Lindane?' said Jeremy when he heard about our tests. 'I remember Lindane. We used to dress the grain with it to kill weevil. We had to, by law.'

'By law? What, there was a MAFF directive?'

'I think so. I can't really remember. Anyway, it was a white powder that we used to chuck in the top of the silo. If it didn't look like it was going to percolate all the way down the vat we used to just turn the pressure up. The dust used to go everywhere.'

Until this moment I had all but forgotten that in the summer of 1984 I spent a fortnight working on the farm at Furneaux. It was harvest time, and Uncle Kit was short-handed. I was seventeen: I'd just won my driving licence at the second attempt after a test involving an improbable number of mini-roundabouts in Slough. Each morning I clapped on a pair of yellow ear defenders and climbed into the cab of a five-ton tractor-trailer combination. My job was to drive exactly parallel to the hopper-arm of a combine-harvester, at exactly 5 mph, for as many hours of the day as were available. (The moment inevitably came when, engrossed by the moving waterfall of grain over my shoulder, I forgot to look forward. I have never forgotten how the veins stood out on Kit's neck as he roared at me in surreal silence from the soundproof cabin of his combine. Our wheels had interlocked; another foot and one of them would have sheared.)

When the trailer was full I towed it to the drier, two miles up the road.

Waiting by the drier while my trailer emptied, I used to stand around by the grain pile at the bottom of the silo, smoking roll-ups in a cloud of dust that almost certainly contained Lindane.

I rang Uncle Kit to confirm what Jeremy had said.

'I don't think it was the law to use Lindane. Although maybe it was some kind of regulation,' he said. 'I don't know, I can't remember. But we certainly used it. Ask Sheriff's, they're the ones who supplied us.'

There was a pause while Kit thought some more. Like Jeremy, he hadn't been in farming for many years.

'I remember you children all playing in the grain in the barns. Those were the days, eh? You couldn't do that any more. Maybe it wasn't such a good idea.'

This was another unwelcome reminiscence. Before collection, the dressed and dried grain was stored in vast heaps in a pair of lovely old beamed barns in the farmyard. Every summer as children, my sisters and brother and I used to be invited down from London to spend the weekend at the farm. At harvest times we rushed to the barns, where we played for hours in those sleek grain-mountains that shifted like quicksand but wouldn't swallow you up. We whooped all over them, dived from the tops, and even tried to bury ourselves in the grain. Now I wondered which of our backsides contained the highest level of Lindane.

I tried to contact Sheriff's, a small family firm based in Royston, but they had been bought out years ago by the Crop Care Group, which had in turn been merged with Profarma Ltd to form Agrovista UK, a subsidiary of Japan's Marubeni Corporation, which was the sixth-largest company in the world with an annual turnover of $17bn. Small family firms didn't really do agrochemicals any more. Eventually I found a former Sheriff's agronomist called Keith Roberts. Kit, he told me, had been right: there was never any legal obligation to apply Lindane. On the other hand, the pressure to use it had been real enough.

'It was probably a contractual obligation,' Keith Roberts explained. 'Those were common enough at the period. The big buyers obviously didn't want weevil introduced into their stock and often insisted on Lindane treatment before buying in grain from the farms. Lindane was certainly approved for use in that way.'

More often than not, what the farmers used against weevil was decided by the chemical firms themselves.

'The reps used to go round the farms and make suggestions about what chemical to apply and how to apply it. The regulations got tougher through the eighties, and the reps are all properly qualified now, but it wasn't like that in those days. Anyone could be a rep. In fact some of them were really just salesmen.'

'So they could have sold Lindane without giving particular instructions about how to handle it?'

'It's possible. Things were different in those days. It's certainly true that a lot of the chemicals we used then would never get to the market-place now. Paraquat, for instance: no chance. Probably not Lindane, either.'

I rang John McLaren-Howard at Biolab once again. He agreed that my time at Furneaux could well have been the source of my contamination. I emailed another pesticides specialist, a GP in the Welsh Borders renowned for her expertise called Sarah Myhill, who agreed with McLaren-Howard.

'Yes – certainly possible,' she replied. 'Also think of wood timber treatments such as Cuprinol.'

There wasn't much doubt in my mind, however: the fortnight of farming at Furneaux in 1984 was now the prime suspect.

I didn't blame my uncles for using Lindane irresponsibly, nor for letting me and my siblings play in the grain-mountains as children. It wasn't just that Lindane was supposed to be safe in those days; I also understood that they belonged to a generation whose attitude to chemicals was entirely different from ours. They grew up in an era when even the case against smoking had yet to be proved, and in the absence of knowledge came a kind of chemical machismo that had never really left them. In the early 1980s a group of English farmers formed the 'Ten Ton Club', which required members to achieve that yield of wheat per hectare. These farmers did not ask what they could do for the land but what the land could do for them; they didn't spare a thought for the possible consequences for the environment, animal welfare or human health. My uncles were never members of the Ten Ton Club but they shared the go-getting attitude of those who were. Agrochemicals were a godsend, one of the great plus-points of modernity that allowed them to participate in an unprecedented grain-farming revolution: the world's grain harvest almost tripled between 1950 and 1990, from 631 million to 1780 million tonnes.

My parents kept the same faith. To them, organic food seemed little more than a marketing man's con trick, a young person's fad that was both expensive and illogically retrograde.

The extent of our generational difference was underscored one summer evening when Melissa and I went over to my parents for dinner. It was hot, and we were laying the table in the garden. Mum had lit a mosquito coil and placed it in the middle of the table. I moved it further away almost without thinking. She rather irritably put it straight back again, after which no-one said anything, and we all sat down to eat in a miasma of insecticidal smoke. I sneaked a look at the packet later on. The active ingredient was d-Allethrin, a synthetic pyrethroid closely related to the sea-lice killer that had cost Johnny Parry his salmon farm. It was also a suspected endocrine disruptor in humans that was proven to be highly toxic to fish.

Underlying her action was an assumption that the mosquito coil was harmless. If such a product was commercially available, she reasoned, then it followed that it had been rigorously tested for health and safety. She was right in a way: of course it shouldn't be possible, in the twenty-first-century West, to put a suspected endocrine disruptor in the family shopping basket without realizing it. But because it shouldn't be possible, she had convinced herself that it *wasn't* possible – and that was a leap of faith that I was no longer able to make.

Her attitude towards her microwave oven was just as revealing. She didn't use it exclusively for cooking, but she was fond enough of it to have assigned it a nickname – she called it her 'Mikey' – and often remarked that she couldn't live without it. Melissa's feelings towards microwaves, by contrast, were downright hostile. Our kitchen was pre-fitted with one: we only ever used it as a plate-warmer. My own feelings were ambivalent. As a lazy bachelor I had been every bit as pleased as my mother still was with the convenience of microwave ovens. But then one of my aunts showed me an article, much photocopied and circulated, suggesting that the intense internal heat produced by microwaves damaged the molecular structure of certain foods, and could drastically diminish their vitamin and nutrient content. Even worse, there appeared to be evidence that cooking with microwaves sometimes created free radicals and other cancer-causing agents, such as d-Nitrosodiethanolamine.

I was sceptical at first. The magazine that published the article, *What Doctors Don't Tell You*, was aimed squarely at hypochondriacs, budding orthorexics and other paranoid obsessives, and obviously had an agenda. Yet some of the article's material could not be ignored. I was surprised to learn that in 1976, following some damning research at the Institute of Radio Technology at Klinsk in Byelorussia, the Soviet Union banned microwave ovens altogether; the ban was not lifted until after Perestroika, a decade later.

'Somebody already sent me that article,' said Mum when I showed her. 'I read it. It was completely unscientific. I threw it away.'

'But what about the Russians?'

'That was a long time ago. I bet they were using some old kind of microwave that isn't around any more.'

I read out some other passages: the article didn't sound unscientific to me. Researchers at Stanford University in California in 1992 discovered that microwaving breast milk caused a considerable decrease in 'anti-infective factors'; a Swiss scientist named Hertel found in 1989 that people fed exclusively on microwaved food experienced a worrying drop in their white blood cell count. But my mother was obdurate.

'It's all rubbish. What we need is a proper *scientific* comparison between microwaved and conventionally cooked foods. Then I might be convinced.'

Her loyalty towards the Mikey was unassailable. The convenience of fast food didn't merely outweigh any possible risks: it nullified them.

She was not the only one to be so seduced. Even Marguerite Patten, the doyenne of home-cooking, thought microwaves were such a boon to the hard-pressed housewife that she accepted the presidency of the Microwave Technologies Association, an oven-manufacturers' trade organization. Melissa's mother's relationship with her microwave was almost as close as my mother's. She spoke cheerfully about 'nuking' food for the family table – which, given the military antecedents of microwave technology, was actually rather appropriate. An offshoot of Allied radar research, the invention dates from 1946 and is usually accredited to Dr Percy Spencer, who in the course of an experiment with a magnetron tube noticed that a bar of chocolate in his pocket had melted. The first appliances, giant contraptions designed for restaurants, were known as 'radaranges'. On the other hand, some historians reckon that a German version of the microwave oven was used earlier by U-boat crews to heat their *Kartoffeln* – in which case the war in the Atlantic had an even greater effect on British eating habits than Hitler and Admiral Dönitz intended. Either way, the microwave oven was a child of the war, just as agro-chemicals and both of our mothers were; and the speed and convenience it represented was a direct dividend of the peace. Perhaps that explained our mothers' blinkered embrace of the modern kitchen's most con-spicuous symbol of progress.

The nutrient depletion of microwaved foods was precisely the sort of issue that would have engaged the attention of Jack Drummond. Britain's mass adoption of the technology – the ownership of microwave ovens rose from 46 per cent of households in 1992 to 87 per cent ten years later

– would have troubled the man who believed that the key to good health was a sound understanding of food and cookery. No doubt he would have had something to say on the matter, but he was murdered in the very year that the US firm, Raytheon, launched the first countertop microwave for use in homes.

His untimely death, I thought darkly, must have been a relief for Raytheon. In the sphere of human nutrition, who else in the West counselled caution in the race to develop technology that affected it? As in the agrochemical sector, the possibility that the integrity of foodstuffs might be dangerously altered was largely ignored in the 1950s. Concerned by 'anomalies' in the behaviour of DDT, Drummond had advocated a 'wide range of tests' on new agrochemicals in his *Chemistry and Food* lecture in 1951. The most that ICI could manage in their tests on Lindane was to observe that it made potatoes taste 'musty'. The precautionary principle should have been applied to the first microwave ovens, too, but apart from in an obscure research laboratory in Byelorussia, it never was. Big business had the bit between its teeth: the rewards of bringing new technology into the home were simply too great. Raytheon was typical. Thanks in part to its pioneering role in the development of microwave ovens, the firm became the twenty-first century's largest missile-maker and the fourth-largest US defence contractor, with revenues approaching $17bn. Money, I was sure, was a key reason for my family's contamination with Lindane and DDT and all the other poisons identified by Biolab. Big businesses like ICI and Geigy and Raytheon had so much to gain from the silencing of their few opponents.

I was not alone in this sinister observation. One day I went to visit a food expert, Professor Michael Crawford of London Metropolitan University. For the past fifteen years he had headed the LMU's Institute of Brain Chemistry and Human Nutrition. He had won a clutch of prestigious prizes for his pioneer research into the effects of poor maternal diet on the development of the foetal brain, and the importance of consuming the right proportions of essential fatty acids. He was one of the country's top exponents of the nutritionist's mantra, 'you are what you eat'. His institute occupied a single floor near the top of an unprepossessing tower block on the Holloway Road in north London. I found his office at the end of a dark linoleum-covered corridor, just past a laboratory where a solitary white-coated student was applying a Bunsen burner to a Meccano-like structure of test tubes, bell-jars and retort stands. The professor was a pleasant man who spoke with a mild Scottish accent. He looked a little like Tony Benn, the socialist politician, but without the pipe.

I was there to question him about chicken. His views on the subject had recently been quoted in a magazine article. Melissa and I had switched to organic chicken many months ago, but Michael Crawford contended, disturbingly, that this was not necessarily a good alternative to the cheap but fatty beasts available in the supermarkets. He was happy now to explain how he had roasted and analysed a bird from a large organic farm in the Home Counties. Its operators had been so confident in the quality of their poultry that they had invited a team from LMU to come and see for themselves.

'In many ways it was an impressive operation,' he said. 'The feed was good. They were doing wonderful things with spent coffee grains, collected from the local Starbucks, and the chickens were certainly free range.'

Sadly, the result was a chicken that still contained only slightly less fat than protein.

'Even organic chickens tend to be overfed. And they are likely to come from a strain specifically bred for weight gain.'

The professor agreed that modern food in general wasn't nearly as healthy as the public thought it was, a state of affairs he blamed squarely on the food manufacturers. It was at this point that I discovered he was a lifelong admirer of Jack Drummond.

'Have you heard of a book called *The Englishman's Food*?' he said. 'It's all in there . . . there's no better account of how the manufacturers have manipulated people's eating habits over the years in the name of profit.'

He was the first fellow Drummond aficionado that I had met. It was like coming across a countryman in an unlikely corner of a foreign land. His interest in Drummond, I discovered, was more than merely professional. His wife had been best friends with one of the daughters of Drummond's friend and protégé, the biochemist Guy Marrian – probably the last Englishman to see Drummond alive. In the 1950s, furthermore, Mrs Crawford had worked as an au pair in Marseilles for the family of one of the prosecutors involved in the murder trial. Although the killings were by then some years old, they were still the subject of speculation in the prosecutor's household.

'My wife told me that he was never very happy about the safety of Gaston Dominici's conviction. With good reason, of course. It was a complete cock-up.'

'You don't think Dominici did it, then?'

'There was certainly something very fishy about the affair. Imagine how different things might have been had Drummond lived.'

'There's a suggestion in France that he was assassinated by the KGB.'

'Really? I don't know about that. But the timing of his death was certainly very . . . shall we say, *convenient* for the food manufacturers.'

'Are you saying that he was bumped off by big business interests?'

The professor considered this, leaning back in his chair and scratching his throat.

'You need to understand the context,' he said. 'The study of human nutrition was still getting off the ground in the 1950s. The establishment didn't like it – so it was suppressed.'

'How so?'

'Why don't I tell you about it over lunch?'

We quit his office and headed for a Thai restaurant above a pub in the Holloway Road where a choice of chicken or beef curry was on offer. We both opted for beef. And then he began to tell me about a friend of Jack

Drummond's called Hugh Sinclair, a don at Oxford in the 1940s, who dreamed of breaking away from the Department of Biochemistry where he worked and setting up an International Centre for the Study of Human Nutrition. Sinclair was well ahead of his time in his conviction, now generally accepted, that heart disease and other degenerative illnesses were caused by a dietary deficiency of essential fatty acids. But Sinclair's dream, despite vociferous support at Whitehall from Drummond, was never realized. Although brilliant, he was ridiculed for his predilection for self-experimentation: on one famous occasion he ate nothing but seal-meat for 100 days.

'Like William Stark and the honey puddings!'

'Exactly so,' Crawford smiled.

Sinclair was courageous, but his personality was abrasive and ill suited to the subtleties of a faculty turf-war. In the end he ruffled the Oxford establishment's feathers so badly that his funding was withdrawn and he was effectively fired. Hans Krebs, the head of the Biochemistry Department, was reputedly so infuriated by Sinclair that he broke up his office with a sledge-hammer.

'Krebs,' I said. 'Any relation to Sir John Krebs, the ex-head of the Food Standards Agency?'

'His father.'

It seemed that the Tom-and-Jerry war between those who wanted to reform food production and apologists for its industrialization had been running for two generations at least. John Krebs had recently resigned from the FSA, where his easy-going attitude towards agro-chemicals and the new technology of Genetic Modification, together with his casual dismissal of the organic food industry, had drawn frequent criticism even in the mainstream press. That unreassuring formulation 'the benefits of eating "x" outweigh the potential disadvantages' was his. He once famously remarked that a cup of coffee contained more carcinogens than the average person ingested from pesticide residues in food in the course of a whole year.

'The FSA's food safety agenda is transparent,' Crawford maintained. 'It's nothing but a smokescreen for industry.'

Sinclair, he explained, was not the only visionary nutritionist whose ambitions were ruthlessly quashed. The successor to the body planned by Sinclair, the British Nutrition Foundation, was established in 1967 as a rigorously independent research institute. But the BNF was 'turned' by the food companies such as Marks and Spencer, Tate and Lyle, and Unilever, who still finance it today. Crawford believed that the 1969 death from a sudden heart attack of the BNF's founder and first director-general, the fat particulate specialist Alastair Frazer, was also suspiciously 'convenient' for big business. The same was true of the Agriculture and Food Research Council, which was closed down in the 1980s: 'the last bastion of the idea that nutrition and health are intimately linked', according to Crawford.

In short, the nutrition movement in Britain was still-born. To this day there is no dedicated faculty of human nutrition at any of Britain's major universities. The topic is still perceived as an upstart newcomer to academia – an interesting but minor subset of biochemistry, at best. Nutritionists are still routinely dismissed as cranks, as Eve Balfour was, or are simply ignored, as Robert McCarrison was before her. It was typical that Dr John McLaren-Howard, the director of Biolab, qualified at the American College of Nutrition – for the very good reason that no heavyweight equivalent exists in Britain. Crawford had himself encountered the old prejudices. He had moved to London Metropolitan University when his original berth at UCL was lost to a funding cut. His nutrition faculty at LMU – surely one of the capital's more obscure centres of academic excellence – was tiny, especially when compared to the vast and far more popular computer studies faculty that occupied two whole floors below him. He showed me the teeming computer rooms with a resigned air, like a man who knew the precariousness of his position. It was only later that I discovered that Crawford was the chairman of the McCarrison Society, a body dedicated to keeping the torch of independent nutrition research aflame.

Crawford's meaning was clear: Drummond's murder was the keystone in a dastardly campaign of corporate suppression, without which the course of nutritional history in Britain might have been entirely different. It was quite a conspiracy theory.

'Did you know that Drummond was planning an updated edition of *The Englishman's Food* when he died?' he said finally. 'Who knows what he intended to put in it. His notes were never found.'

'Are you suggesting they were stolen?'

'Maybe – or maybe he never found the time to write them. In the end a colleague of his from the Ministry of Food, Dot Hollingsworth, revised the book herself on behalf of his executors. She was most interesting on the subject. It's a shame you can't talk to her – she didn't die all that long ago.'

'Yes, but . . . do you really think he was *assassinated* by big business interests?'

'I don't know,' the professor shrugged. 'You'd have to find out. But it wouldn't surprise me in the least.'

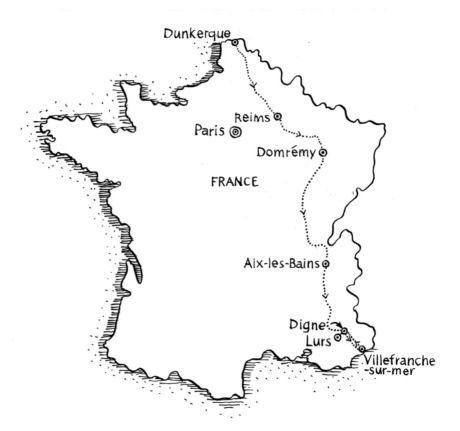

The Drummonds' Route 27th July – 4th August 1952

Dunkerque

Reims

Paris

Domrémy

FRANCE

Aix-les-Bains

Digne

Lurs

Villefranche
-sur-mer

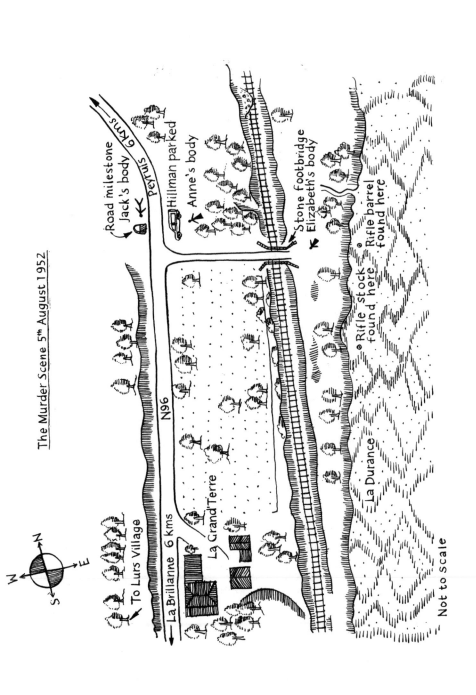

The Murder Scene 5th August 1952

Not to scale

To Lurs Village
La Brillanne   6 kms
N96
La Grand'Terre
La Durance

Road milestone
Jack's body
Peyruis   6 kms
Hillman parked
Anne's body
Stone footbridge
Elizabeth's body
Rifle stock found here
Rifle barrel found here

N
W
E
S

Chapter 5

The Murders

'What the general public thought of canned meats in the 1860s can
be judged from the name given by the Navy to the products
produced by the newly established canning factory at the
Victualling Yard at Deptford. They called this meat "Sweet Fanny
Adams" . . . The name has been immortalized as a result of a
notorious murder which took place in 1867, when a woman named
Fanny Adams was killed at Alton in Hampshire, her body
afterwards being hacked into small pieces. Her murderer, Frederick
Baker, was hanged in Winchester Gaol on Christmas Eve of that
year. The morbid humour of the sailors at Portsmouth soon traced a
connection between this murder and the canned meat being turned
out at the factory at Deptford. It is one of the few cases where the
victim rather than the murderer has achieved immortality.'

The Englishman's Food

The mystery surrounding the Drummond murders had intrigued me
when I first heard about it in Forcalquier, but I was driven forward now
by something more powerful than mere curiosity. I already knew that big
business, in collusion with the political and military establishment of the
1950s, was responsible for the chemical contamination of my family. If
Michael Crawford was right, then the one man who might have prevented this was killed not by Gaston Dominici but by the same powerful
alliance of interests. Proving this would be personally and professionally

satisfying. It might even rekindle the British public's forgotten interest in my nutritional hero, perhaps opening the way for a timely reappraisal of the lessons Drummond once taught, and the salvation of his reputation. Best of all, of course, was the possibility of finding someone specific to blame for the chemical impurities in our bodies. If the Drummonds were indeed the victims of contract killers, who knew where the money-trail might lead? And so it was with an almost missionary zeal that I bought a clutch of the most recently published French books on the murders, and with the help of a Collins-Robert dictionary open on one knee, set about turning myself into an expert on the Dominici Affair.

The most talked-about French murder mystery of the twentieth century began in an ordinary way. According to the orthodox version of the killings, the reason for the Drummonds' presence in France in the first place was nothing more interesting than a relaxing family holiday. Tourism was undoubtedly one explanation for their trip. Drummond was an ardent Francophile who had visited the country many times before, and who had a passion for French food. He was one of the earliest British members of the International Wine and Food Society, the world's first and most respected diner's club founded in 1933 by the French connoisseur André L. Simon. In Nottingham, Drummond was the society's chief evangelist: when he moved there he quickly became a pillar of its local branch. According to his colleague Frank Young, Drummond's civilizing influence was a light in the darkness of Nottingham, 'an industrial Midland city where much more than lovely old buildings had been swept away under the torrent of wealth which poured from the textile mills in the previous century, and where the arts and gracious ways of living had been swamped to such an extent that they had not yet completely recovered'. In the 1940s and 1950s any epicurean would have welcomed the opportunity to swap the austerity of Britain's post-war kitchen for the markets and restaurants of France.

Drummond, moreover, was recovering from a bout of ill-health in 1952. At the beginning of the year he had suffered a cerebral haemorrhage. His heart had been murmuring, too, a recurrence of a malady that had troubled him all his life. By July, however, he was feeling much better. His daughter's school had broken up for the summer holidays, so when Professor Guy Marrian, a biochemist colleague from UCL days and one of his best friends, invited the Drummonds to stay at a rented villa at Villefranche-sur-mer, near Nice, he readily accepted.

They set out from their home at Spencer House in Nuthall, near Nottingham, in an olive-green Hillman estate – a shooting brake, as such cars were called then – on 25 July. The car, and its licence plate NNK 686, were soon to achieve an unexpected notoriety. In contemporary newspaper photographs it now seems almost impossibly quaint. With its un-aerodynamic curves and oddly elongated body, it looks the sort of machine that a grown-up Noddy might have driven.

They caught a ferry from Dover to Dunkerque on 27 July. From there they drove slowly down the eastern side of France, stopping for the night at various scenic spots along the way – Reims, Domrémy, Aix-les-Bains. On the face of things they looked and behaved just like any other English family on holiday. Elizabeth was an only child of above-average intelligence, and her parents adored her. It was typical of them to allow her to set some of the itinerary for their drive south. Domrémy, for instance, was her idea. On 29 July she sent a postcard from there to her favourite schoolteacher in Nottingham, a Miss Hancock, who didn't receive it until after the sender's death. 'We are having a lovely time in France,' she wrote. 'We have just visited the birth-place of Joan of Arc. It is quite nice weather but rather cold.'

They stopped for the night at the Grand Hotel in Digne in the foothills of the Alps on Friday 1 August, 60 miles short of their final destination. Here Elizabeth spotted a poster advertising a *charlottade*, a type of bull-run, which was to take place there in three days' time. The family was expected chez Marrian the following day; Elizabeth made her doting father promise to bring her back to see the bull-run on Monday.

The weekend at the Marrians' went well. The parents were able to relax after their long car journey, and the Marrian daughters, Valerie and Jacqueline, twenty and twenty-three respectively, were charmed by the ten-year-old Elizabeth. The Drummonds set off for Digne again very early on the morning of 4 August, with Jack at the wheel. They left their luggage, passports and most of their money behind with the Marrians for safe-keeping, as the excursion was only for the day. The *charlottade* took place in the late afternoon. Several spectators later recalled seeing the family in the crowd. Afterwards they had an early supper at a local hotel, L'Ermitage, before leaving Digne again in the car.

They did not take the direct route back south to Villefranche, the tortuous Route Napoléon up which they had travelled that morning, but instead headed west along the Durance valley in the direction of Marseilles. Their decision has never been explained; some newsmen speculated that Anne Drummond had been alarmed by the twists and turns of the old road, and had requested they return by a less vertiginous route, no matter how much longer it might be. For whatever reason, the family trundled westwards on Route Nationale 96; and as darkness fell (or so the newsmen again speculated), they decided to stop and camp, intending to complete their journey the following morning. At last they spotted a likely site, a grassy flat spot near a small stone bridge leading down to the river, not far from the village of Lurs. There was a picturesque farmhouse near by called La Grand'Terre. This was the home of a family of Franco-Italian peasant farmers called Dominici – Gaston, his wife Marie, their son Gustave, Gustave's wife Yvette, and baby Alain, the future defender of the family name.

Much of what happened next is still hotly disputed. There were no witnesses other than the Dominicis, and their evidence was a tangled mass of contradictions, half-truths and downright lies. However, it seems likely that the men of the family were drunk when the Drummonds arrived. The Basses-Alpes region was poorly irrigated in the 1950s, so farmers had to water their crops and orchards according to a strict monthly rota. It had been the Dominicis' turn that day, and it was their custom to celebrate the completion of the *arrosage* with copious amounts of wine. Unfortunately they forgot to turn off the irrigation taps, causing an embankment to collapse onto the railway line that formed one edge of the property. La Grand'Terre was a world away from the steely efficiency of the agricultural revolution going on elsewhere. The Dominicis had no need for mechanization or agrochemicals. Their little patch of ground had been farmed in the same old way for years. The railway line was blocked, but there was no emergency, for it was seldom used, and the appropriate authorities had been warned. It would be all right to wait until the morning to clear it.

The Drummonds had had a long day too, and turned in early. Elizabeth slept in the back of the Hillman, with the adults on camp-beds just outside. Before bed, Anne and Elizabeth may or may not have knocked on the farmhouse door to ask for a bucket of fresh water: the Dominicis contradicted themselves over this. Either way, they must have known that there was a family of foreigners camping at the end of their field. The Hillman was less than 200 yards away and clearly visible from the house.

At 1.10 a.m., seven shots resounded across the valley. If the Dominicis had nothing to do with the murders as they at first claimed, their reaction to this disturbance was strange – the first of many actions that led to a widespread assumption of their guilt. None of them, they insisted, got up to investigate or even looked out of the window in the direction of the campsite. Gaston told the police that he thought it was poachers shooting rabbits, and that he had rolled over and gone back to sleep. It was not until dawn that a passing motorcyclist, Jean-Marie Olivier, was flagged down by Gustave, who announced that he had found three dead bodies and that Olivier should fetch the gendarmes.

The police investigation, led by Commissaire Edmond Sébeille of Marseilles, was a disaster from the start. Arriving late on the scene, the police did nothing to secure the area, where a large number of sightseers and local journalists had already gathered, wandering at will and destroying potentially crucial forensic evidence on the ground. According to Roger Lachat of the *Dauphiné Libéré*, it was the journalists and not the police who first identified the victims, because they searched the car before the gendarmes did.

The investigators did agree on some things, though, and it wasn't long before they had pieced together a version of what had happened. The motive for the murders was probably not robbery. The interior of the Hillman was an indescribable mess, which made it hard to know what might be missing, yet nothing obvious seemed to have been taken, notably a 5000 franc banknote. Anne's body was nearest to the car, and although it had been moved it had clearly not been moved far. She had been shot while lying down, presumably in her sleep. It followed therefore that she had been killed first. Jack's body, covered over with a camp-bed by persons unknown, lay across the road. But a small fragment of flesh from his finger was found on the bumper of the car, suggesting that he had not died immediately. The investigators deduced that he had struggled with the killer, or killers, before staggering across the road where he died.

Elizabeth's death was more of a puzzle. Her corpse was found 77 metres away, down a path over the bridge that crossed the railway line. There was little blood found by her body, despite the fact that her head had been staved in, leading some to surmise that she, too, had been moved. Although barefoot, her feet seemed strangely unblemished by the stony ground across which she must have run. But the consensus of opinion was that she had witnessed her parents' deaths from the car where she had been sleeping, escaped through a side-door, and fled for her life. The stonework of the bridge was found to be freshly chipped, perhaps by a bullet, suggesting that the gunman had fired after her and missed. Sébeille was convinced that she had died where she now lay.

The murder weapon was quickly recovered from a pool in the river where it had been tossed by the killer: a battered Rock-Ola US army carbine held together with wire and a piece of bicycle. A splinter of wood found by Elizabeth's head matched a gap in the shattered stock, proving that this was the instrument with which she had been finished off. The Rock-Ola was a kind of firearm that abounded in the region, abandoned or traded for food by US infantrymen as their liberation of Europe rolled northwards in the summer of 1944. It was a well-known model, nicknamed the 'Little Darlin'' by GIs; an estimated 6000 of them were issued to American forces serving in France. Amazingly, no-one thought to test the carbine for fingerprints until it had been passed around among the curious hordes, by which time it was too late. However, it seemed probable that the gun belonged to one or other of the Dominici family. When Gaston's elder son Clovis was shown the weapon, he turned white and fell to his knees.

Until this moment, no-one had suspected that the Dominicis were involved. Their behaviour until then had seemed innocent enough. Both Gaston and Gustave repeatedly told those who asked, and even those who did not, of their horror and outrage at the crime on their doorstep. They were loud in their opinion that a deserter from the Foreign Legion – an early police suspect, later ruled out – would prove to be the culprit. Gustave posed for press photographs and seemed almost proud of his discovery of the bodies and his promptitude in alerting the authorities. Gaston showed visiting journalists around his property and appeared to go out of his way to assist the police. Later, indeed, he was to claim that it was he who had spotted and turned in the shard of wood from the rifle butt.

The sorry news didn't take long to reach London, where it instantly made the front pages. The authorities seem to have been careless about informing the next-of-kin before the murders were reported. In Drummond's case, of course, there were no next-of-kin; but for Constance Wilbraham, Anne's aged mother, the blow was so brutal that she immediately suffered a stroke and remained paralysed until her death in 1959, unable to move anything but an arm. The nearest Jack had to a relative was a godson, Mike Austin-Smith, whose father had been brought up almost next door to Jack back in the early days in Charlton.

Mike was dead, but his eighty-year-old sister, Silvia, was still alive. In fact she lived less than a mile from where Melissa and I did in west London.

I went to see her and her 91-year-old husband, Graham Tharpe, in their cluttered flat, where we sat down together over mugs of tea at her kitchen table. Jack, she affirmed, had adored her and Mike. She remembered a kind, friendly man who always had time for them. As children, they called him 'Uncle Jack'.

'Family was important to Jack because he himself had none. Looking back I realize that we Austin-Smiths mattered more to him than I thought at the time. We were his surrogate family.'

The Austin-Smiths still saw Drummond regularly as teenagers in the 1930s, and had reason to respect his unusual expertise in nutrition.

'We had an Airedale terrier,' Silvia recalled, 'and there was something wrong with its top and bottom lips. Jack took one look and diagnosed vitamin A deficiency. It was my first instruction in the practical application of cod liver oil.'

His promotion to the Ministry of Food in 1940 filled them with pride.

'He was tall and good-looking, and his new job was so glamorous and important. But we weren't at all surprised because we all thought he was brilliant. He was always fascinated by food, and so passionate about it.'

She covered her eyes as she recalled the moment when she learned of the murders, from an *Evening Standard* billboard spotted while walking down the Strand.

'It was unbearable. I was pregnant with my first child at the time, which made it even harder to cope. I think I blotted it from my mind. It was just too horrible to deal with.'

Elizabeth's death hit her hardest. When Silvia married in 1949, Elizabeth had been her bridesmaid. She remembered the ten-year-old as 'a dear little girl, and highly intelligent. Jack was besotted with her.'

She doodled viciously on a notepad as she spoke, the tight little circles thickly overlaying one other. It was chastening to watch – a reminder that the Drummonds were not just characters in a murder mystery but had once been a part of real people's lives. Silvia's feelings were raw, even after so many years.

'I know it's ridiculous,' she went on, 'but I still feel guilty somehow that I wasn't there to stop those bastards. That poor, poor little girl . . . she was such a sweet thing.'

She said she still dreamed of Elizabeth in her last moments, scrambling in her pyjamas from her hiding place in the back of the car and scampering frantically down the dark path to the riverbank. The dream always ended there; she said she never dwelled on what happened when the path ran out and the killer with the empty rifle caught up with her.

Silvia explained how the funeral arrangements were left to her brother, who flew out to France at once to help the Marrians, although it was her decision to have the Drummonds buried there.

'Mike was for bringing the bodies back to England. But he rang me because he wasn't sure, and I said no, leave them in France. I told him, Jack loved France.'

(She was right about this. Many of his pre-war experiments on vitamin B deficiency were conducted in France. In 1937 he delivered a paper to the eleventh Congrès International de la Société scientifique d'hygiène alimentaire on the relationship between vitamins B and E in the diet and the reproduction system. Some of his experiments involved the controlled starvation of human volunteers, a technique for which he could not get permission in London. Drummond was suitably grateful, and maintained a friendly working relationship with the scientific community in Paris. Of the many international honours conferred upon him after the war, it was his degree from the University of Paris that pleased him the most.)

The ceremony at Forcalquier took place on 7 August, just two days after they died. The tremendous heat of Provence made any further delay inadvisable.

'What about the Dominicis? Do you think they did it?'

'Mike always thought so. Then again, no-one was ever really sure. I remember speaking to Mike on the telephone before the funeral, and he was shocked even then at the shambles the police had made of things. He went to look at the murder site, and there were people roaming all over it. But in the end, Mike was pretty sure that they'd got the right man. He met the Dominicis and thought they were "shifty".'

'You know about the conspiracy theories in France?'

'The KGB theory you mean. Yes, I heard about that. There was supposed to be a hit squad from East Germany or somewhere, but I'm sure it's not true. If the killers were Germans I'm sure they would have been more efficient.'

'Did he have any enemies that you were aware of?'

'Jack? Good Lord, no. He was the most likeable man imaginable.'

'Within the food or chemical industries, for example.'

'I never heard anything like that.'

Hers was the standard explanation of the murders – the one so doggedly pursued by Commissaire Sébeille. It was obviously many years since she had reflected on the possibility that the Drummonds had been murdered by contract killers, and it seemed unkind to push it. I felt awkward enough already, blundering about in the attic of her memories. On her doorstep as I was leaving, however, she held me back.

'There is one other thing,' she said. 'On the evening before the Drummonds left for France, a friend dropped in on them at Spencer House. I probably shouldn't be telling you this, but . . . he told me later that Jack had been drinking heavily. He noticed because it was so unusual: Jack was never a big drinker. So maybe you're right. Maybe he did have enemies. Maybe he secretly knew that there was trouble ahead.'

Sébeille and his team were soon under immense pressure to catch and convict a culprit. The columns of the Parisian press fulminated against the nation's shame. 'All France is roused in horror and indignation at this monstrous triple crime,' said an editorial in *France-Soir*. 'It is a blot on France's honour as a host . . . It is essential that the Drummonds should be avenged and that justice should be done. The reputation of France is at stake.' This might well have been true, for the world's press had descended on the Basses-Alpes in unprecedented numbers. The funeral itself was a big media event. Forcalquier had not known a scene like it since 1944, when ten gendarmes were ceremoniously shot by the Germans. Shops and businesses closed their shutters as three mule-drawn hearses made their way from the hospital chapel to the cemetery. The town's entire population, about 2000 people, turned out to pay their respects, and were joined by a further 2000 from the neighbouring region. The hearses were followed by schoolgirls wearing white dresses and carrying wreathes; hymns were sung by a Protestant choir specially bussed in from Nice. The British contingent was led by Mike Austin-Smith, the Marrian family and the British Consul-General from Marseilles.

The tightly packed crowds surged down the cemetery staircases, trampling on graves and standing on tombstones for a better view. There was silence for the graveside oration delivered by the Mayor of Forcalquier, Léon Espariat. Some of his audience sobbed. 'Sir Jack Drummond and his family will sleep their last sleep in the soil of France, which they loved so much, in the soil which is also theirs because so many British soldiers shed their blood with their French comrades to defend it … the whole French nation is united with the British people in their grief.'

His words were merely the first in a series of emotional testimonials that now poured forth, both in France and at home.

'Tell the people of Britain that we shall never forget these three graves,' the Vice-Prefect of Forcalquier, Gustave Degrave, told the reporter from the *Daily Express*.

Sébeille, certain that he would soon solve the crime, told the press that 'the murder weapon will speak'. But as time went by it became clear that his early confidence was misplaced. The murder weapon did not speak. The rustic inhabitants of La Grand'Terre were by now the prime suspects, but however suggestive Clovis's reaction to the sight of the Rock-Ola might have been, the Commissaire also knew that it proved nothing. Travelling with his team of investigators from house to house, Sébeille was met with what he described as 'a wall of silence'. No-one, it seemed, knew anything, and the true ownership of the gun was never satisfactorily established. The investigation was eventually to drag on for fifteen months, a delay for which the Commissaire was attacked by the press on both sides of the Channel. Fleet Street nicknamed him 'the Maigret of Marseilles', after the protagonist of the novels of Georges Simenon, which were then much in vogue. He resembled Maigret slightly, with his stylish trenchcoat and air of studied nonchalance. The French, meanwhile, called him 'Commissaire Tourne-en-rond' – Superintendent Round-in-circles.

There were good reasons for the recalcitrance he encountered among the locals. The Lurs region in the 1950s was a poor place, populated by tough peasant farmers still haunted by the memory of the war. The maquis, the mainly Communist Resistance, had been strong here, but there were also many who had collaborated with the Germans. There were many scores to settle after the Liberation, and the maquis had not been disarmed. Some had formed themselves into vicious gangs bent on plunder and extortion. The region was widely believed to be full of hidden treasure. Quantities of gold, pounds sterling or forged French banknotes had been parachuted to the Resistance. Rumours persisted that the war-chest had been raided by the maquis, or by criminals masquerading as such. Mysterious shootings in the night were therefore commonplace throughout the area, not only as the war ended but for years afterwards, too. The bullet-riddled body of a photographer, André Gras, was found beneath the football stadium at Forcalquier in 1944. A young hairdresser, Mademoiselle Collette, was murdered at Les Mées, as were an old couple who kept a tobacconist's shop at Mallefougasse. The old Mayor of Peyruis, Monsieur Musy, and the local judge, Monsieur Stain, were both assassinated. At a farm at Pierrerue, an entire family was killed. Even more notorious were the killings at Château de Paillerol, just across the river from Lurs. Monsieur and Madame Cartier, who lived there, were shot one night by a gang of burglars. Then the police commissioner sent up from Nice to investigate, Jean Stigny, was himself murdered and his corpse dumped in a ditch just opposite La Grand'Terre. To survive in such a fearful environment, the locals naturally kept themselves to themselves: it was simply safer not to get involved. Perhaps fear explained the Dominicis' failure to react to the gunshots on their doorstep.

Sébeille had another problem. The wider public's imagination was so gripped that, by the time of the trial in November 1954, his team had received some 5000 tip-offs relating to the affair. It was impossible not to sympathize with the poor policemen who were obliged to follow up every lead. Even the British police, who were never involved in the investigation on the ground, were inundated with obfuscating information. I visited the Public Records Office at Kew to look up the old case files. Many of the letters they contained were, frankly, mad. One, dated November 1952, was from a spiritualist in Tunbridge Wells called Lady Knollys, who wrote to say that Anne Drummond had come to her in a dream to reveal the murderer's identity: a local psychopath (nameless, naturally) who had blackmailed the Dominicis into taking the blame. There were a student of 'electro-magnetic radiation' from Isère called LeGros, offering the divining services of a special pendulum of his own invention; a medium from Johannesburg who wrote to say that he had seen 'a man standing on a railway track holding a hammer'; and someone from Liverpool claiming to have proof that the culprit was one 'Jim Phelan, a communist'. Best of all was an anonymous letter blaming the IRA. The killings, its author explained, were to avenge the Irish National Dance Team who had recently been prevented from singing their national anthem, 'The Soldier's Song', at the Nice Folk Festival – an insult that became unforgivable when the Union Jack was flown as the troupe began their dance routine.

The whole world, it seemed, was hooked. In 1955, Orson Welles made a twenty-six-minute film about the murders, *The Tragedy of Lurs*. It was one of a seven-part inaugural documentary series for the new British television channel, ITV.

'No writer could imagine characters like these Dominici,' Welles declared to the press. 'You have to see them to believe it.'

The film was left unfinished and never broadcast: Welles had failed to apply for an official permit before filming began, and was then refused permission to export it following pressure by Marcel Massot, the local MP.

'It would be scandalous if the publicity given to this sad affair were prolonged outside France by television,' Massot complained. 'From moral considerations and from the point of view of French propaganda, the exportation of such a film should not be tolerated.'

The film was never made commercially available in Britain, but it was in America. I obtained a copy on the Internet and had it converted from the US PAL format in a specialist shop off the Strand. Then I watched, fascinated, as Welles himself interviewed character witnesses and Dominici family members on the actual site of the murders. Shot in the grainy black and white of the period, the piece was moody and brilliant, its pervasive sense of menace oddly enhanced by the fact that it was just a fragment.

As Welles observed, the Dominicis were the inhabitants of a vanishing pre-industrial world. Gaston Dominici was the very image of the peasant patriarch. A moustachioed man of seventy-six with a face as gnarled as the stick he leaned upon, he was fiercely proud of his independence and the fact that he had built up his farming business from scratch. He was fond of the bottle and irascible when drunk; he ruled over his extended family with a discipline that could be despotic. At the same time he was a generous host who always had time for strangers, inviting them in for a chat and a drink of his home-made wine. He presented himself as the salt of the earth, a good citizen, a patriot who loved his land and his country. Indeed, he described himself in patois as *'un homme franc z'et loyal'* – a straightforward and dependable man – so often that it later became a catchphrase of the trial. On the other hand, there were plenty of detractors who reckoned his outward appearance concealed an interior of rat-like cunning.

Commissaire Sébeille did not give up. One after the other, the Dominicis were pulled in for interview at the Palais de Justice in Digne. Gustave's interrogation lasted for three days. This was undoubtedly hard for the family – 'When will this Calvary end?' his feisty wife, Yvette, was once heard to cry – although the experience hardly amounted to the police brutality that was later alleged. Sébeille was convinced that at the very least they knew more than they were letting on – particularly the feckless Gustave, whom a passing motorist had seen darting out from behind the Hillman a few hours after the murders. Under pressure, Gustave at one point admitted that it was he who had moved the body of Anne Drummond – looking, he said, for spent bullet-casings that might help the police investigation. In fact several bullet-casings, which might well have been interesting to a ballistics expert, were later found to have disappeared from the scene. Gustave later changed his story; he ducked and weaved and lied as though he had been born to it. Yvette was caught lying, too. There was also something suspicious about Roger Perrin, Gustave's sixteen-year-old nephew, who lived a few miles away, but who had been at La Grand'Terre on the evening of the crime. He claimed he had gone home before the murders, and that at five o'clock the following morning he had been collecting milk from a farmer called Puisant. The alibi was idiotic: the police checked and discovered that Puisant had died six months previously. Sébeille was sure the boy was hiding something, but still he could prove nothing.

With a solution continuing to elude Sébeille, speculation soon began to fill the void. Even his colleagues within the police had ideas of their own. Michael Crawford, I discovered, was not the first person to suspect that big business interests were involved. In an internal report of August 1952, a divisional superintendent called Harzig told his superiors that he believed the murders to be 'an episode in the secret struggle between pharmaceutical corporations' – a suspicion prompted by Drummond's position at the time as a director of Boots. This, however, was the closest anyone ever came to the big business theory. Far more popular at the time was the idea, repeated forty-five years later by the investigative journalist William Reymond, that Drummond was some kind of British government spy, and the murders a murky episode of the Cold War. This suggestion first surfaced in the Communist press, particularly *La Marseillaise* and *L'Humanité*. The assassins were, according to one's political predilections, Russians, Americans or Germans. The enemy agents had been looking for 'a document'; they had followed the family all across France, waiting for an opportune moment to strike; La Grand'Terre had been cynically chosen so that the police would suspect the farm's innocent inhabitants and be thrown off the scent.

The testimony of a traffic policeman named Émile Marquet threw fuel on the fire. Marquet was on duty in Digne on the evening of the murders. At about 8.15 p.m. he observed a car with British number-plates pull up outside L'Ermitage, the town-centre hotel where the Drummonds had been dining an hour before. The driver – '1.80m, svelte, about 30, in a t-shirt and white trousers' – asked Marquet if he had seen another English car passing that way. When Marquet affirmed that he had, the driver asked what direction it had taken. Then he went inside, leaving his companion, a 'woman in black', standing by the car. A quarter of an hour later – the time taken, say, to place an international phone call – he emerged from the hotel at a run, jumped into the car with the woman in black, and sped off in the direction taken by the Drummonds an hour before. It looked as though the Drummonds were being followed. But why, and by whom? The couple were never identified or traced. Were these, perhaps, the emissaries of some British chemicals corporation bent on assassination?

Some held that Drummond had been an agent for the SOE, the London-based Special Operations Executive that took over many of the functions of MI6 during the war, and that had supplied and worked alongside the maquis from 1940 onwards. Seven years on, it was suggested, Drummond had been sent by London to settle accounts with the ex-maquisards, or perhaps to demand the return of stolen parachute gold. Such speculation was not confined to the French. In London, the *Daily Express* advanced a sensational theory that the Dominicis were part of a Communist gun-trafficking ring. La Grand'Terre, the *Express* explained, was a staging post in an underground trail that led to Marseilles, from where guns could be smuggled to the left-wing insurgents of the FLN in Algeria. A convoy of arms had been due to leave the farm on 5 August; the Drummonds had simply been in the wrong place at the wrong time. Gaston's superior, the *Express* went on – a mysterious figure called 'Esteban' – had ordered Gaston to tell the English holidaymakers to go and find somewhere else to camp. When Jack Drummond obstinately refused, Esteban ordered Gaston and Gustave to kill the family. Terrified and too compromised to argue, the Dominicis did as they were told. Another version of the same story held that the Dominicis were the guardians of a secret arms dump, to be kept in readiness for the Red Army when it marched west.

The Dominicis were, in fact, staunch Communists. This was nothing unusual: 30 per cent of the French had voted Communist even before the war, and in many parts of the country, Lurs included, the percentage was now considerably greater. Like all good Communists, the Dominicis had also assisted the maquis during the war. A cell of fighters had been established on the Ganagobie plain, which towered over the Durance valley and the Dominici farmstead below: Gaston was said to have supplied the cell with food. With the armistice still just seven years old, the line between the Communists and the glorious Resistance was understandably thin in the public's perception. The moment the direction of Sébeille's suspicions became known, therefore, the Communist press flew to the family's defence. The allegations against the Dominicis, the papers claimed, amounted to a politically motivated attack on the reputation of the noble Resistance itself. As an outsider from Marseilles, Sébeille was obliged to tread very carefully indeed. Veiled warnings came from as far away as Paris that he was not to stir the pot too hard, for fear of creating a southern political imbroglio.

The machinations of the local Communist Party added to Sébeille's woes. Shortly after the murders, a senior Communist Party official from the capital toured all the farms of the region to encourage – or perhaps order – the locals not to cooperate with the police investigation. Meanwhile, Sébeille could not help but notice the unexpected visitors who kept arriving at the Dominici home, including the municipal councillors of Lurs and the local heads of the Communist Party. The meetings they held in the kitchen of La Grand'Terre were closed, and no word of what was said at them was ever forthcoming. A new piece of graffiti, swiftly replicated across the region, served as a reminder of what the Commissaire was up against: *'L'URSS domine ici'*. This clever double-entendre – it meant 'The USSR runs things around here', but sounded like 'Lurs Dominci' – was interpreted locally as another coded admonition to the police.

Curiously, it was gossip among members of the local Communist Party that led to Sébeille's eventual breakthrough. It seemed that Gustave had confided to a family friend, Paul Maillet, that Elizabeth had still been alive when he found her. Why Maillet let this confidence slip was itself the subject of intense media speculation. A railway linesman like Gustave's older brother Clovis, Maillet was also the head of the local Communist Party cell with a proven Resistance background. When the police swept the area for clues after the murders, they paid a visit to Maillet's house and found a clutch of Sten-guns hidden in an oven. Interviewed by Orson Welles three years later, he was still insisting that Gustave was guilty. Maillet wore an enormous beret and spoke with a stubby pipe clamped permanently between his teeth, making his Provençal accent even more impenetrable than usual. He also winked constantly, an unfortunate nervous tick for someone supposedly telling the truth. He was pure vaudeville: the only thing missing was a string of onions and a bicycle. No wonder Welles was fascinated.

Gustave was brought in for questioning once again. Confronted by Maillet, he was forced to confess: Elizabeth had indeed still been just alive when he found her body. He had got up very early, he explained, in order to inspect the landslide on the railway line, and heard her groaning in the undergrowth. Yet neither he nor any other member of his family had done a thing to help the girl, or had even gone near her – on the grounds, Gustave claimed, that he was frightened of leaving incriminating footprints. He was later charged with failure to assist a person in danger, and imprisoned for two months. Under mounting pressure, Gustave at last appeared to crack – and blurted that it was not he but his father who was the killer. He was later to retract this startling confession, only to repeat it again. By the time of his father's trial, he had retracted and repeated it no less than a dozen times. Nothing he said could ever really be trusted. Nevertheless, the charge that he had abandoned a wounded ten-year-old was enough to cause the Communist Party to forsake his family's cause. It was one thing to protect the reputation of an honest working-class family, but quite another if Sébeille had been right after all to suspect them. The tide had turned against the Dominicis. From now on they were on their own.

Sébeille, scenting an arrest at last, now focused his attention on Gaston. Confronted with news of his younger brother Gustave's allegation, Clovis at first denied but then admitted that he, too, was convinced that his father was the culprit. One evening at La Grand'Terre, he told Sébeille, Gaston had been drunk and abusive towards his wife, Marie, a wizened old lady whom he habitually addressed as 'the Sardine'. Clovis now relayed the following Provençal outburst from the lips of his father: '*Lei ai fa péta toute très. Si nin fau faie péta inca un, lou faraï péta.*' Sébeille understood this to mean: 'I've already killed three people. If I have to kill another one, I will.'

It was not the first indication that the old man was prone to bouts of drunken rage. Gustave's accusation began to look as though it might be true. Gaston was brought in for questioning once again. After a lull of several months in the press, what was by now known as the Dominici Affair again became headline news. Gaston was the new arch-villain. He was dubbed the Wild Boar of La Grand'Terre, the Horrible Assassin, the Monster of the Basses-Alpes. In London, the entire Dominici family were now being described as 'beasts in shoes'. To begin with, Gaston furiously denied the accusations made by his sons, whom he denounced as 'pigs'. He even shouted out that they were the murderers, not he. Locked up overnight, however, he appeared to have a change of heart, and confessed.

The confession brought fresh problems for Sébeille. The details of Gaston's story kept changing. At first he explained that he had gone out to inspect the landslide on the railway line, taking his rifle with him – he 'didn't know why' – and had been jumped on by Drummond, who 'must have taken me for a marauder'. He had killed the Englishman in self-defence, and then Anne and Elizabeth because they were witnesses. But when asked to repeat this version of events later on, Gaston told a different story. The motive now was sexual – very explicitly so. 'Passing the English campsite en route to the landslide, I saw the man sleeping and the woman in the process of taking off her dress,' he told his incredulous interviewers. 'I looked at the woman. I suddenly wanted to fuck her. She saw me but she didn't seem frightened. I grabbed her crotch. She didn't react. I didn't hesitate, I got my cock out. She lay down on the ground. We fucked . . . then the husband woke up. He came towards me. I took up the rifle. He tried to take it from me . . . the shot went off by accident.'

This was the stuff of an old man's fantasy. The sexual motive seemed preposterous: Gaston was seventy-six in 1952, and Anne a matronly forty-eight. The suggestion that she would willingly fornicate with a stranger while her husband and daughter slept yards away was clearly ridiculous. There was no forensic evidence of sexual assault, and the bullet holes in Anne's corpse suggested she had been shot while asleep. From what dark recess of Gaston's mind had the story sprung? Sébeille noted that it was common knowledge that Gaston hadn't shared the Sardine's bed in years. Yet Gaston not only stuck with his new story but embellished it at each repetition, adding more and more salacious detail each time. It was as though he took a perverse pleasure in his shocking self-incrimination. It was also clear that he didn't believe a word of what he was saying. More than once he explained that he was only confessing because he wanted to save the reputation of his family. It began to look uncomfortably as though he had calculated that the police would never leave his family alone, and that it would therefore be best for all of them if he took the blame. He might even have reasoned to himself that the courts were more likely to be lenient with him than with the younger men of the clan.

In an effort to clarify what had really happened, Sébeille decided to make Gaston participate in a reconstruction of the crime. The first attempt had to be postponed when the date of this event was leaked to the media. The police arrived at La Grand'Terre with Gaston to find more than a hundred cars parked along the road. The place swarmed with the press and curious members of the public, who had covered the murder-site with bunches of flowers. They tried again the following day. Gaston, pursued by gendarmes, policemen, magistrates and photographers, marched through the motions of the crime without showing the slightest emotion. He even seemed to be enjoying his performance. When the moment came to replay the struggle with Drummond, he gave the policeman playing him a real punch on the nose.

The mood changed when Gaston was ordered to re-enact his pursuit of Elizabeth. As the circus crossed the little railway bridge he astonished everybody by breaking away from his attendants and hurling himself towards the parapet. A genuine suicide attempt, or another *coup de théâtre*? It was never clear. Whatever his motivation, he was only narrowly prevented from falling 25 feet onto the railway line. After that he baulked at continuing with the reconstruction – the part that dealt with the death of Elizabeth. His reticence was noted. Was he so horrified by what he had done to the girl that he now couldn't bear to be reminded of it? Or was he unwilling because he wasn't responsible for this aspect of the triple crime?

Either way, Gaston's performance was enough to convince the accompanying magistrates of his guilt. The moment the reconstruction was over, the old man was led up the steps of a police van specially furnished with a table and chair, where he was charged and made to sign the committal papers. It was November 1953, fifteen months after the Drummonds had died. The stage was set for what the French press were already calling the trial of the century.

The old man's chances didn't look good. My chances of standing up the Crawford theory didn't look very good, either. Apart from the unsubstantiated suspicions of Superintendent Harzig, and the unresolved identity of the English couple reported by the traffic policeman, Émile Marquet, I could find nothing to support the idea of corporate assassination. By contrast, the more I learned about the behaviour of the Dominicis in the wake of the murders, the more convinced I became that they were implicated. The fire of conspiracy theory began to burn less brightly within me; I worried that the Dominici Affair was nothing but an enormous red herring, and that Drummond's murder had no connection at all with agrochemicals or my family's contamination.

I pushed on, though, and began to search hard for a retired reporter who had been at the trial. I was amazed to find one eventually almost under my nose. In the early 1990s Ronald Payne and I had worked closely together on the features desk of the *European*, the now defunct newspaper launched by the ill-fated tycoon Robert Maxwell. I hadn't known then that in 1952 he was one of the *Daily Telegraph*'s correspondents in Paris, from where he was dispatched to report on the affair.

I went to see Ronnie at his cottage near Minster Lovell in the Oxfordshire Cotswolds. Now in his late seventies, Ronnie was an acknowledged authority on terrorism. He had been appointed as the *Telegraph*'s Middle East correspondent by 1954, when he was sent back to

France specifically in order to cover the trial. Blessed with that capacity for reinvention that all the best journalists have, he had recently scored an unlikely success with the publication of a slim volume called *One Hundred Ways to Live with a Cat Addict*, a reference to his wife Celia Haddon, the author of a long-running weekly newspaper column about pets.

He led me into the garden, limping slightly from a helicopter crash long ago in Oman. The house was on a high, treeless plateau and surrounded on all sides by huge, newly ploughed fields. A solitary cock pheasant – a frequent visitor from the wood on the far horizon, Ronnie said – strutted proprietorially along the edge of a carefully tended flowerbed. He and Celia hadn't lived here for very long and were proud of their new house, although to my over-sensitized eyes the place looked fearfully vulnerable to contamination from crop-sprays.

The cottage had once been part of a farmhouse, and the attached farmyard was still in operation. A monster tractor stood idle in the corner, guarding a barn that I could easily believe was filled to the rafters with dangerous, endocrine-disrupting chemicals. When Ronnie mentioned that the whole area had once been a part of the royal hunting forest of Wychwood even in his lifetime, I realized that he was living at the centre of a desolate monument to the hedge-rooting, tree-hacking agricultural policies of the 1950s. I was careful not to mention it, but it seemed to me as though the plateau had been scorched by some almighty unseen hand, and Ronnie's garden, a tiny oasis in a desert of mud, was all that had survived.

He described the famous trial at Digne as a 'glorious farce'. The little town seethed with journalists from around the world – 175 of them in all. Ronnie remembered overhearing the public prosecutor, a bombastic little man called Louis Sabatier, rehearsing his opening speech to the jury before a mirror in the neighbouring room at the local hotel. He was an excellent mimic and hadn't forgotten what he'd overheard.

'*Mesdames et messieurs,*' he began, trying not to giggle as he puffed out his chest like the pheasant in the garden, *'je vous affirme* solennellement *que ce crime méchant est une honte pour la France . . . une honte!'*

Five thousand people turned up to watch on the first day and had to be turned away. The courthouse was the smallest in the whole of France. Ronnie was one of the lucky ones: in those days journalists were considered almost as an integral part of the trial process, and the more important among them were guaranteed a place. The unlucky ones left outside had to make do with a mobile press room, a specially adapted bus equipped with multiple telephone lines, which was more usually used to cover presidential visits or national events like the Tour de France. There was no press gallery in the courtroom. Instead the newsmen and women were invited to squeeze in wherever they could. Back inside the cottage, Ronnie produced a scrapbook filled with photographs, including one of him squatting in the very centre of the packed courtroom.

When the court went into recess for lunch each day, the journalists repaired en masse to one of the bars in Digne's central boulevard, where, in time-honoured tradition, they interviewed each other. As a correspondent from London, Ronnie was much sought out by his French counterparts for his views on the guilt or otherwise of the accused. In retrospect it was one of the earliest trials-by-media in history. There was much criticism later that the press had interfered materially in the course of justice. It was said that the enormous number of journalists in the courtroom, and the constant popping of flashbulbs and whirring of camera motors that attended their presence, had intimidated the witnesses. The Dominici trial was to become a French legal landmark: photographers were excluded by law from courtrooms ever afterwards.

It was true that the press did not distinguish themselves by their behaviour during the affair. They had hampered Sébeille throughout his investigation, notably with their interference with potentially crucial evidence on the morning the murders were discovered. Since then they had harried Sébeille wherever he went, and alternately befriended or spied on the Dominicis themselves. Some had even hidden themselves in an outhouse of La Grand'Terre in the hope of overhearing some juicy piece of new evidence. In the shameless scramble for exclusivity, the worst interferer was perhaps Jacques Chapus of *France-Soir*, who fabricated an entire travelogue purportedly written by Elizabeth. Her supposed notebook even included a description of the evening she was killed. Chapus's report was picked up by rivals and republished everywhere, obfuscating Sébeille's enquiries and causing untold emotional pain among family and friends of the Drummonds back in Britain. During the trial Chapus was called to testify to a conversation he had held with Gaston, but even then he said nothing to correct the false impression he had created.

The trial lasted ten days, during which the French justice system did not excel itself either. Under the constitution of the short-lived Fourth Republic, juries comprised seven members of the public plus a senior member of the judiciary, the President of the Court. Unlike in Britain, where juries are enjoined to reach a verdict through private and independent debate, in France in 1954 their decision was directed by the Court President. In this case the President was a Niçois named Marcel Bousquet, who since the Liberation had directed all the great trials of collaborators at Marseilles. Despite his experience he was accused of bias and incompetence from the outset, especially in the British press. The trial had been delayed for too long. The pressure from Paris to reach a speedy conclusion had not abated. Even today, defenders of Gaston Dominici suggest darkly that he was a hapless pawn in a game of international politics, and that the notion of justice was sacrificed on the altar of Anglo-French relations.

Bousquet's job was certainly not easy. First, there was a language problem. Gaston's first language was Provençal, not French, and he was often unable to understand what the court was talking about. Either his vocabulary was too limited, or else he assigned his own meanings to words that Bousquet assumed were in common usage. In *Mythologies*, a collection of essays published in 1957, the famous semiologist Roland

Barthes described the entire process as a 'trial of words . . . [there was] a complete misunderstanding of syntax'.

'*Gaston Dominici, êtes-vous allé au pont?*' Gaston was asked at one point. ('Gaston Dominici, did you go to the bridge?')

'*Allée? Il n'y a pas d'allée,*' he replied. '*Je le sais, j'y suis été.*' ('Alley? There is no alley. I should know, I've been there.')

Language was not the only gap between the worlds of the lawyers and the Dominicis. As the family members were brought one by one before the court, it became evident that Bousquet was no better equipped to make sense of the lies, evasions and contradictions in their stories than the police had been. Gaston's performance, by contrast, was astounding. If he felt intimidated by his situation he never showed it.

'If am convicted,' he said grandly, 'I don't want to be guillotined, I want to be burned like Joan of Arc, exiled like Napoleon, or crucified like Christ.'

He maintained his innocence with such stoutness that even the cynics in the audience wavered. His defence was based on a counter-accusation that some other member of his family was guilty of the murders. But even with the spotlight of the world's attention upon him, he refused to say which one.

His exchanges with his family members were naturally tense. Gustave's appearance in the witness box was particularly extraordinary. He was apparently so in awe of his father that in his presence he was unable to bring himself to repeat the allegation that had led to Gaston's arrest in the first place. He wriggled pathetically, desperate to justify himself.

'It's true that I denounced my father, but only because I was frightened they might say that I'd killed the girl,' he said at one point. 'In any case, I wasn't the first one to accuse him.'

He told the court that he thought perhaps Elizabeth's parents had killed the girl, and that such things happened all the time.

'It is impossible to imagine someone more cynical, more ignoble or more stupid,' one journalist wrote.

Gustave's filial loyalty was so utterly misplaced that even Gaston held his head in his hands.

'Saying that I'm innocent isn't enough!' the old man shouted from the dock. 'I've told you that I'll forgive you if you tell the truth. Tell them!'

But it was too much for his feeble-minded son.

'I've already told the truth,' Gustave mumbled. 'I don't know anything.'

The press looked on, mesmerized by this strange family squabble, throughout which not one Dominici ever expressed any compassion or remorse for the murdered English. Gaston's real character seemed exposed early on during testimony from the Marrian parents. Three months after the killings they had visited the murder-site in order to meditate on the deaths of their friends. Gaston, they said, had 'popped up like a tour-guide' to show them around. The Marrians didn't realize who the old man was at the time; he finished his guided tour by pestering them for a tip.

Bousquet was out of his depth. Over and over he was bamboozled into fruitless debate over irrelevant detail while failing to focus on what mattered. One journalist described the trial as a kind of surreal ballet, with a theme of denial that recurred like some musical counterpoint: 'First theme: we've never seen the Rock-Ola rifle. Second theme: it was Clovis, not Gustave, who denounced Gaston first. Third theme: the confessions of both Gaston and Gustave were down to police brutality.' The trial frequently descended into chaos, with various members of the Dominici family shouting at each other across the courtroom with such force that Bousquet struggled to regain control.

There was another sensational moment during Clovis's testimony. For two years the family had denied ever having seen the Rock-Ola rifle. Gaston now pointed furiously at Clovis and said, 'You're the one who looked after the gun. It was you who patched it up – I saw you do it!' The outburst prompted a renewed explosion of shouting, not only between all the Dominicis present but also between the astounded lawyers of the prosecution and defence. This might have been a turning point in the trial, yet once again Bousquet failed to press home the advantage. Instead of letting the exchange run its course he chose to suspend the hearing to restore order to his courtroom. As one writer commented, he seemed to be a man who preferred order to the truth. Either way, Gaston's faux pas was never referred to again – an amazing oversight that on its own might justify the description of the trial as a farce. As the court broke up after Clovis's testimony, one of the Dominicis – no-one was ever able to tell which – was heard to yell above the hubbub: 'Liars! We are all of us liars!' As one disquieted journalist later wrote, these tortured words sounded like a shriek from some inner circle of Hell.

Fifty years on, Ronnie Payne was still convinced that the Dominicis were guilty. The only ambiguity, he reckoned, was whether Gaston, Gustave or Roger Perrin had pulled the trigger. He thought Gustave could well have persuaded Gaston to plead guilty on the grounds that the court was less likely to condemn an old man to the guillotine.

'In the end, one or other of the Dominicis was definitely guilty – guilty as sin,' Ronnie concluded.

'But what was the motive?' I asked. 'It surely wasn't robbery. There was a large banknote on view in the car. A thief would have taken it.'

'Sex, probably,' Ronnie shrugged. 'In my experience it very often is.'

'But Gaston was seventy-six! And Anne was, what, forty-eight? And she wasn't exactly a looker.'

'True,' Ronnie laughed, 'but he was drunk – and you should have seen the Sardine.'

I was forced to add Ronnie to the growing list of those who thought Commissaire Sébeille had essentially got it right. He had no time at all for the idea that the KGB were responsible: 'real French horseshit', he called it. I explained Michael Crawford's reasons for thinking agrochemical or food manufacturing interests were responsible. Ronnie doubted it very much, although he conceded that in the context of the Cold War anything was possible.

'There was some talk before the trial about the murders being connected somehow with a nearby chemicals factory. But the factory wasn't actually that close by, and it was certainly never mentioned in the trial.'

However doubtful Gaston's claim of a full-blown sexual encounter with Anne, I had to agree that prurience could have played a role, particularly where the other two Dominici suspects were concerned. This was the theory of the journalist Jean-Charles Deniau, whose 2004 book, *DOMINICI – It was a Family Affair!*, was written as a riposte to the KGB hypothesis embraced by William Reymond. In Deniau's scenario, Gustave and the teenage Roger, drunk after the celebration of the *arrosage*, had gone out to spy on the English campers, perhaps taking the gun with them in order to scare them. They were just out to have a bit of fun at the foreigners' expense. But the Peeping Toms were caught by Jack, there was an altercation, and everything went horribly wrong. After the shootings they panicked and returned to the house, where Gaston took charge. According to Deniau, it could have been he who went back out to the campsite, discovered Elizabeth, and finished her off with the rifle butt before disposing of the weapon. It was as plausible an explanation as anything else I had read or heard.

Deniau had one further possible explanation for why Gaston was prepared to protect Gustave and his grandson Roger – particularly Roger. While under arrest he told police constantly that his confession was a 'sin of love', and that he was making it only to 'save the honour of his nineteen grandchildren'. In the course of the investigation, however, a twist emerged that was worthy of the darkest Pagnol plot. It was whispered that Roger, son of his daughter Germaine, was in fact also his son; and that Roger not only knew it, but also that Gaston would go to any length to prevent this shameful fact from becoming public. This, it was said, explained why Roger behaved so strangely in the witness box, smiling and laughing to himself like he was half-demented.

However unsatisfactory the trial might have been, its outcome was unequivocal: Gaston was found guilty on 28 November and sentenced to the guillotine. But soon afterwards he let it be known from his prison cell that he had fresh information that would lead to the real killer. His lawyers seized on this and applied for a stay of execution. Public disquiet at the way the trial had been handled prompted the Garde des Sceaux in Paris, the equivalent of the Lord Chancellor's office, to grant the stay pending another investigation. As one of Gaston's lawyers remarked: 'The trial may be over, but the Dominici Affair is just beginning.'

The new enquiry, led by the crack Paris investigator Charles Chenevier, got under way in 1955 – and went nowhere. The 'fresh information' promised by Gaston amounted to a conversation he claimed to have overheard between Gustave and Yvette that suggested that it was Roger Perrin who had moved the body of Elizabeth. If Gaston's intention during the trial had been to protect his grandson, he had now changed his mind. His new claim was impossible to prove, however. And Chenevier and his team had another problem: they had to contend not only with the famous 'wall of silence' among the Basses-Alpes locals, but also with the non-co-operation of the provincial judiciary, who felt professionally insulted by this intervention from the capital. Chenevier, well aware of how under-interrogated Roger had been both before and during the trial, had intended to question him closely. But the official permission he required was denied him by the Digne magistrates. Such obstructionism turned the new enquiry into a fiasco and further fuelled the speculation that the murders were the subject of an official cover-up. Although convinced of Roger Perrin's complicity, Chenevier and his team were forced to return to Paris. 'We need proof, not probabilities,' the judge in charge intoned. In March 1956, three and half years after the Drummonds were murdered, the second enquiry was dismissed.

Yet the conspiracy theory gossip did not go away, any more than the uneasy feeling among the public that the case against Gaston had not been satisfactorily proved. Signing the old man's final death warrant must have looked politically risky to the authorities in Paris. The President, René Coty, quickly commuted Gaston's sentence to life in prison. Coty was succeeded in 1959 by Charles de Gaulle, who ordered the old man's release on humanitarian grounds, reputedly following pressure from his wife, Yvonne. De Gaulle stopped short of issuing a presidential pardon, though, and ignored Gaston's written request for a retrial. Gaston was a weak old man by the time of his release, hardly recognizable to those who had seen him perform so robustly in court. He died in a hospice at Digne in 1965 aged eighty-nine, still protesting his innocence.

Yvonne de Gaulle was not the only one interested in absolving Gaston. In south London in 1959, two associates of the Dominici family tricked their way into the old people's home of Constance Wilbraham, Anne's tragically paralysed mother. Posing as law students, they questioned her at length and returned to France claiming that she had forgiven her daughter's murderer on her deathbed. There was still enough life left in the old lady to launch legal proceedings, however. Ever since the murders she had kept a photograph of Elizabeth on her bedside table, fondling it occasionally with her one good arm. Every year on 22 March, Elizabeth's birthday, her room was filled with flowers sent by friends, relatives and well-wishers. 'I am dying of bitterness,' she reportedly said before she really did die, 'with nothing but bitterness in my heart.'

There was one other curious postscript to the tragedy. Even before the trial ended the Drummonds' Hillman was sold, apparently to the Louis Tussaud waxworks museum in Blackpool. In the summer of 1954, in a tented show on the Promenade, it became the centrepiece of a mock-up of the famous crime scene. The show included a pair of mannequin corpses topped with badly moulded waxwork heads. It must have made an effective advertisement for the nascent domestic tourist industry: who would want to go camping in France after a show like that? I rang the museum to see what had happened to the heads, and indeed to the Hillman, but the archivist there had no record of either. In fact he wasn't even convinced that the show had taken place in Blackpool, and suggested I try Morecambe, just up the coast.

I decided then that I was wasting my time. According to one account I had read, the car had been exhibited not at Blackpool or Morecambe but on the seafront at Brighton. Nor was it quite clear why or how the car was released from police custody so prematurely. During the trial, Marcel Bousquet proposed that the assembly adjourn to the police compound for an inspection of the car, only to be told that it was no longer there; the court was obliged to make do with a substitute car specially brought up from a garage in Nice. The Hillman is now almost certainly lost, while a single photograph taken in the Blackpool rain, lifted from the archives of *Paris Match* and poorly reproduced on a French Dominici Affair website, is the only evidence that the waxwork heads ever existed.

Chapter 6

The Other Drummond

'One of the most foolish fallacies concerning "tinned" foods is that
they are liable to cause cancer. It is impossible to say how this idea
arose but it is a reasonable conjecture that it originated from an
attempt to account for the increase in the prevalence of the disease
during the past forty or fifty years. So far as scientific grounds for
the belief are concerned one could with equal justification blame the
increasing use of the telephone or the decline in popularity of straw
hats.'

The Englishman's Food

The Crawford conspiracy theory was already crumbling at the edges.
Now, however, I discovered something that caused it to disintegrate
entirely, and that turned everything I thought I knew about Drummond
on its head. His directorship at the Boots Pure Drug Company in
Nottingham was the sticking point. I had presumed that the job was a
cosy sinecure, a part-time position accepted in lieu of something worthy
of his talents; it was, perhaps, something to tide him over until his Tory
friends regained their political footing in London. I couldn't have been
more wrong.

My mistake was to think of Boots as the kind of firm that it is today: a
humdrum chain of high-street dispensaries where the nation buys its
soap and toothbrushes. The company's nineteenth-century origins were
in retailing, it was true, but in Drummond's time its whole direction and

purpose were radically different. Here was the crunch: in the late 1940s, Boots was at the forefront of the race to develop agrochemicals, with a research department that in some respects rivaled ICI's. Research into new agricultural, horticultural and veterinary products was a pet interest of the chairman, Lord Trent, who had taken over from his father, the company founder Jesse Boot, in 1931. In 1935 an 'experimental station' was established in the gardens of Lord Trent's private residence, Lenton House outside Nottingham. Before long almost the whole of the grounds was taken over by greenhouses, much to the chagrin of Lady Trent. New horticultural laboratories were added in 1947. The company's agricultural division was also greatly enlarged after the war. By 1952, when Drummond died, Boots was farming some 4500 acres in England and Scotland purely for experimental purposes.

That was not all. The directorship taken up by Drummond was not some honorary non-executive post, as I'd thought, but the important and very much hands-on position of Director of Research; and he seemed to have thrown himself into his new job with the dedication for which he was famous. Transcripts of Boots' sixty-second Annual General Meeting in the summer of 1950 showed that sales for that year had beaten all previous records, notably in the farms and gardens department, where sales had risen by more than 26 per cent. Lord Trent explicitly credited Jack Drummond with this success. New agrochemical products placed on the market as the direct result of the research department's work, the chairman proudly announced, included Cornox, a 'selective weed killer', and Turk-e-san, a drug for treating blackhead, a fatal liver disease in turkeys. Drummond, he added, was to be rewarded for his labours with a new research institute at Nottingham.

I looked up Turk-e-san and found that it had been taken off the market many years ago, when it was replaced by Emtryl – which itself was banned by the European Union in 2003 over fears that it was carcinogenic. There is currently no known veterinary treatment for blackhead in turkeys. Then I looked up Cornox. It was based on a Boots-developed formula called 2,4-DP, or Dichlorprop: one of the chlorine-based phenoxy family of hormone weed-killers that were chemically descended from ICI's wartime invention, MCPA.

The formula, which became a world best-seller for Boots, is still listed by the Pesticides Action Network as a 'Bad Actor' chemical. A known marine pollutant, it is also one of the commonest chlorine-derived contaminants found in the modern human body. Its long-term human health effects are uncertain, but are thought to include peripheral damage to the human nerve system and possibly cancer. In 2003, continuing concerns over the lack of data about Dichlorprop led the EU to force those companies using it in their products to either prove that it had no adverse effect on human health, or else to surrender their licence to sell. Daunted by the cost of the necessary laboratory tests, the manufacturers backed off. In 2003 in the UK, 135 agricultural and 81 garden products were withdrawn from sale. More than 70 of the garden products – including Boots Nettle and Bramble Weed-killer, the modern household version of Cornox – were based on Dichlorprop.

That Drummond might have been responsible for the development of Cornox was confounding news. This was the man who advocated the exhaustive testing of new agrochemicals in a prestigious public lecture shortly before his death. Yet here was hard evidence that he did not practise what he preached. Boots had not tested Dichlorprop any more exhaustively than ICI had tested MCPA or Lindane. It followed, furthermore, that Drummond could not possibly have been assassinated by big business interests, because by 1952 he represented those interests. The sagacious author of *The Englishman's Food* had effectively become the chemical farmer's friend. On the face of things Drummond's move to Boots, and what that company's research laboratory produced under his direction, amounted to a spectacular abandonment of the principles and beliefs that had governed his whole professional life. What on earth was he thinking?

I backtracked, looking for clues. Rereading the obituaries archived at the Royal Society, I saw that I was not alone in my mystification. Various explanations were offered for Drummond's move to Nottingham, the most charitable of which was that he hoped to try to influence the new industry from the inside. One writer suggested that he wanted to 'diminish the barriers that inevitably exist between industrial research workers and their academic counterparts'. No doubt there was some truth in this. Bridging the gap between opposing interests was one of his special talents. At Nottingham he became a founder member and the first chairman of the Fine Chemicals Group of the Society of Chemical Industry, whose motto, 'Where science meets industry', spoke for itself.

The commoner explanation was also the least kind: that he needed the money. No doubt this also played a part. He had been offered a senior job that carried a salary of 'not less than £4000' according to a gossip columnist at the time – the equivalent of about £100,000 today. Then as now, academics were not highly paid, whether they were in the employ of the government or not. Drummond, who was fifty-four in 1945, had given his life to academia and had complained – privately, to friends – that he never made any serious money. From 1942 he also had a young daughter's education to pay for. Yet I struggled with the idea that Drummond was nothing more than a sell-out. It didn't fit with what I knew of his manifest passion and commitment to the principles of sound public nutrition. I clung to the shipwreck of an idea that there was a hidden but ethically purer reason for his extraordinary career change.

I rang Peter Campbell, the octogenarian Emeritus Professor of Biochemistry at UCL. He had not forgotten Drummond, whose move to Nottingham he described as 'very curious'. In those days, he explained, it was simply not done for distinguished academics to go off to work for industry – a trend, he said, that did not get under way until about 1960.

'Drummond cut himself off entirely. His choice of Boots was curious, too. Boots never did any decent research.'

Drummond did not bother to keep a foot planted in his old camp. In 1946 he resigned his Chair of Biochemistry, which he had held *in absentia* throughout the war, and turned his back on academia for ever. His collected bibliography ran to an impressive 183 separate publications. Articles, lectures and serious academic papers had poured from his pen in earlier years, most of them with titles like 'The absorption of copper during the digestion of vegetables artificially coloured with copper salts' (1925) or 'The Properties of halibut-liver oil' (1933). In some years, as many as thirteen different publications had appeared under his name. Even in 1941, probably the busiest year of his life, he found time to publish a paper entitled 'Sesame cake and antler growth'. From 1946, however, the publications began to dwindle, and after 1948 they dried up completely. Barring the odd guest appearance – such as his *Chemistry and Food* lecture to the Chemical Council in 1951 – his withdrawal from the debate on public nutrition with which he had been engaged since 1914 was total.

Campbell first met Drummond in 1940, when he went to the Ministry of Food to offer him his services as a biochemist. The offer was turned down, and Campbell spent most of the war involved in the manufacture of radar tubes, but when he arrived at UCL in 1946 he found the legacy of the popular former department head everywhere about him. As he pointed out, Drummond's old university had not forgotten him. A fellowship was set up after his death, and is still funding research; a Drummond Prize was founded in 1973, and is awarded each year to promising students of biochemistry.

'He was much missed by his former colleagues,' Campbell recalled. 'They were puzzled. They assumed he would come back to UCL after the war. He would have been welcomed there with open arms. Working for Boots seemed a bit like going over to the enemy.'

The enemy's lair was still in Nottingham. I wrote to them, asking if I could visit their plant. They answered politely but firmly in the negative, citing reasons of post-9/11 security. So I rang their press office to enquire if I might at least examine the company archives, but was told that these too were closed to the public.

'What about Sir Jack Drummond, then? Can you tell me anything about him?'

'Never heard of him,' said the press officer.

'He was your Director of Research until 1952.'

'Was he now? I'm afraid I've only been with the company for eighteen months. Perhaps you should speak to the archive department.'

I spoke to an archivist, a longtime employee who had at least heard of Drummond. She faxed me an obituary notice from the October 1952 edition of *The Bee*, the Boots staff magazine. The overblown language this was written in was interesting: 'Gifted and gallant gentleman; charming and gracious lady; happy and loving child,' it read. 'There was not to be one last rose of summer; with one swift gust, the cruel wind of Fate scattered the petals of two lovely blossoms and snapped off a sweetly-opening bud.' But apart from the revelation that Drummond had been a 'very keen gardener' – something he had learned to do, perhaps, at the elbow of his adoptive father, George Spinks – it added nothing at all to what I had already gleaned elsewhere.

I rang the archive department back, convinced that they must have more information than this about Drummond and his research department activities. Boots were proud of the fact that they had been in business since 1849. There was even a separate section on their website entitled 'Our Heritage'.

'Sorry, but no,' the archivist replied. 'I'm afraid this department was only set up ten years ago, and the records we inherited were pretty patchy.'

'So the obituary is all you've got?'

'I'm afraid so.'

'What about anecdotally? Is Jack Drummond a part of company lore? What does he mean to you personally, for example?'

'Well, nothing, basically.'

'Does Boots perhaps have some kind of prepared statement on his murder? I know I'm not the first journalist to ask about it.'

'You'd have to ask the press office about that.'

It was hopeless: Boots' institutional memory had been deleted as thoroughly as if someone had pushed the wrong button on a computer.

I tried another tack and discovered that Sir Gordon Hobday, who took over from Drummond as Director of Research in 1952 at the age of thirty-six, was still alive and in retirement near Nottingham. I wrote to him, and he invited me to tea. Hobday was a scientist of distinction and a Boots company legend. He worked on penicillin with Alexander Fleming, and directed the team that invented Brufen, better known today as Ibuprofen. Research on the pain-killer, originally intended for the treatment of rheumatoid arthritis, began at Boots in 1952 and took ten years to perfect. Today, sales of the compound are worth almost half a billion pounds in Britain alone. Hobday went on to become Boots' chairman, the Chancellor of Nottingham University, and Lord Lieutenant of the county.

My interview was an uncomfortable one. He and his American wife lived in a secluded bungalow just north of Nottingham in the grounds of Newstead Abbey Park, the one-time family home of Lord Byron. On my drive northwards he phoned to warn that a dead body had just been found in the lake down by the abbey; the police were treating it as suspicious, so I should expect to be questioned at the gates to the park. The motorway traffic was so bad that I arrived three hours late, upon which he and his wife invited me to stay for supper. They lived in a bungalow deep within the park in a dank and sunless wood. We were discussing the Drummond murders and the rather unnerving coincidence of this new one, when our talk was interrupted by ghostly floating music, the source of which could not immediately be pinpointed. Sir Gordon looked under the table. Lady Hobday looked under the sideboard. I jumped up and was about to inspect the inside of a hostess tea trolley when I realized the music was coming from my pocket. I had accidentally pressed the play button on my voice recorder: we were listening to an old and unloved tape of Janááek that I had snatched up for recording over as I was leaving London.

I didn't expect the old scientist to much like my suggestion that the chemists of his generation had been less than methodical when it came to testing new products, Dichlorprop in particular. But I was surprised even so by the vehemence of his defence.

'It is impossible to test anything conclusively. Look at that television,' he said, pointing testily at a set in the corner. 'It's bombarding you with all sorts of radio waves all the time. But can you prove they're not harming you? Of course you can't. Everything is a potential risk. Life is a risky business.'

When developing new products, he explained, scientists invariably considered what was known as the 'therapeutic ratio'. The test they applied was deceptively simple: if the potential benefits of a new product were deemed to outweigh its potential risks, then development went ahead.

'But that means scientists are regulated by no-one but themselves,' I protested, 'and it means testing products on humans!'

'Of course! What else are we supposed to do? There's no substitute for putting a product in the marketplace and seeing how it performs, you know. Certainly not rats and mice in a laboratory.'

Hobday's faith in the empiric principle was unshakeable. He even defended the notorious drug Thalidomide, conceding only that the makers were 'a bit slow to withdraw it from the market' once its side-effects were discovered. I knew a bit about those side-effects. There had been a student in my year at university whose wrists began at her shoulder-blades, and who gamely made light of her disability by insisting on rolling her own cigarettes. Thalidomide was made by the West German pharmaceutical firm Grünenthal, and administered as a treatment for insomnia and morning sickness in pregnant women from 1957 to 1961. It caused severe birth defects in 15,000 mostly German and British children, only about half of whom survived their first year of life. A court trial revealed that the proper tests, notably those involving pregnant animals, had never been done. In some cases the results were faked. The Thalidomide affair is still seen as the classic example of corporate malpractice in the pharmaceutical industry. I had certainly never heard it defended before.

Scientists, I understood, were obliged all the time by their work to take ethical decisions of the most enormous consequence, the kind of decisions that the rest of us seldom have to grapple with in life. This was the inventor of Ibuprofen sitting opposite me, not some corrupt or greedy businessman. I felt like Justin, the ingenuous hero of John Le Carré's *The Constant Gardener*, floundering in a world that defied straightforward moral categorization. An episode sprang to mind where he travels to Berlin to meet Birgit, a hard-headed anti-pharmaceuticals campaigner and former associate of his murdered wife. 'This does not signify that Dypraxa is a bad drug, Justin,' she tells him. 'Dypraxa is a very good drug that has not completed its trials. Not all doctors can be seduced, not all pharmaceutical companies are careless and greedy . . . The modern pharmaceutical industry is only sixty-five years old. It has good men and women, it has achieved social miracles, but its collective conscience is not developed.'

Hobday knew Drummond well. His daughter went to school with Elizabeth, and he was a part of the small Boots delegation that flew to France to attend the funeral. (Many more Boots people attended a memorial service in Nottingham a few weeks later.) But beyond a remark that he had found Drummond personally 'delightful', he was not very forthcoming about the man he replaced. I sensed that he was wary of my motives for coming to interview him; he seemed to become more reticent as our discussion on the ethics of scientific research became more heated. Drummond had been dead for half a century, yet it was as if the two scientists were closing ranks. When I tried to steer the conversation back to Dichlorprop, he waved the subject away. Drummond's work at Boots, he emphasized, extended well beyond agrochemicals: he had also been a committed enthusiast for new remedies for tropical diseases.

'He was a good man – an altruist,' he told me firmly. 'In fact, between you and me, he wasn't a very good Director of Research. Finding cures for tropical diseases was all very well, but there was never any money in it. We never had the distribution networks to market such products abroad.'

When Hobday took over from Drummond, he explained, almost the first thing he did was to pull the plug on all his predecessor's tropical disease research programmes, and to switch to more commercial projects like Brufen.

'So how did he get the job?'

'He was appointed by the board in the usual way,' Hobday shrugged.

'But why? Wasn't it unusual to appoint an outsider like Drummond to such a key position?'

'I suppose it was a bit of a surprise,' said Hobday, considering this. 'The normal thing would have been to fill the job internally, and there were plenty of suitable candidates. But Drummond had other qualities. His reputation, for example: very useful when it came to raising funds for development projects. And his colleagues never bore any resentment towards him. He was too well liked.'

I had done some research before my Nottingham visit. Despite rising sales and Drummond's contribution to the success of the farms and gardens department, Boots overall was in deep financial trouble after the war. Materials and manpower were in short supply, and maintenance and other costs had rocketed. Two new share issues had to be launched in the early 1950s to pay off an enormous overdraft. Boots was a business like any other, and in the economic depression of the post-war it had been forced to adapt, or die. No private company could afford to be guided by altruism in such an environment. In 1952 Boots opened their first 'super store', the beginning of the transformation of the company into the mass-market, high-street chain familiar in Britain today. The super store immediately drew protests from the traditionalists of the Pharmaceutical Society on the grounds that it was 'debasing the image of pharmacy'. That dispute simmered until 1965, when the Pharmaceutical Society again tried to control what Boots could or couldn't sell through a vote at their

Annual General Meeting. Boots fought them in the High Court, arguing that the Pharmaceutical Society had no legal right to restrain the free development of trade, and won. I had heard an echo of this old confrontation in my telephone conversation with Peter Campbell, whose grandfather had been a pharmacist. As a student he had once wondered aloud whether he, too, should specialize in pharmaceutics. 'Don't do that,' his grandfather told him. 'It's all been ruined by Boots. They're more interested in selling handbags these days.'

(The transformation of Boots was part of a sea-change in the chemical and pharmaceutical industry that has so far proved permanent. No major private firm is engaged these days in the Third World tropical disease research once pursued by Drummond. Researchers are instead focused on finding medicines to treat what the industry calls 'American diseases' – diabetes, heart disease, cancer – because the American market is the only one large enough to allow the manufacturers to recoup the spiralling costs of new drug development. With around 17 million Americans now suffering from diabetes, treatment of disorders relating to it is naturally one of the biggest growth areas. There are currently ten separate anti-diabetes drugs either undergoing late-stage trials or awaiting regulatory approval: Arxxant, Byetta, Denagliptin, Exubera, Galida, Galvus, Januvia, Liraglutide, Pargluva and Saxagliptin.

One of the main reasons that development costs have spiralled is that drug firms are required to test their new products more exhaustively than ever before. Regulations were tightened dramatically after the Thalidomide scandal of 1961. The irony is that the American diseases the firms hope to treat are frequently related to diet and obesity – a problem partly caused by the cheapness of food, which was the result of the industrialization of farming, which was only made possible by the agrochemical innovation for which the same firms were responsible in the first place. ICI, who enriched themselves by selling Lindane and MCPA to the world for half a century, are now profiting all over again by marketing cures for the indirect effects of those products. AstraZeneca, the modern incarnation of ICI, is responsible for the new diabetes drug Galida; potential sales are expected to be in the region of $2bn a year.)

It was true that Drummond brought his own qualities to the Boots boardroom table, but whatever Hobday said, his appointment was still a mysterious one from a commercial point of view. The sort of person the company really needed to lead the research department in the difficult years after the war was a sure-fire money-maker, not an altruistic ex-government adviser with limited experience of business. I was convinced that I was still missing a vital piece of the jigsaw, and that the truth behind Drummond's move to Boots was somehow hidden from me.

The day after my strange supper with the Hobdays – which was followed by an equally strange night in a Nottingham motel full of model train enthusiasts who had congregated there for an annual convention – I drove out to Nuthall to inspect Spencer House. The building was large and white and set among lawns behind mellow brick walls. It had pretty arched windows and its date of construction, 1833, set into the brickwork around the back. Beyond the walls was a scrap of meadow where Elizabeth's pony, Frisky, had once lived. It was a country gentleman's house, although it was clear that the environs were not what they had been in Drummond's day. Nuthall had expanded hugely since the 1950s, while a quarter of a mile away across a field of kale, traffic roared along the M1 bypass. I rang the doorbell, hoping for some titbit of information about the Drummonds, or perhaps even for an invitation to come inside, but there was no-one at home.

I thought a lot about Gordon Hobday's therapeutic ratio on the long and rainy drive back to London. Its implications were startling. There was nothing wrong with the principle – provided that scientists exercised God-like wisdom and judgement when they regulated themselves. I couldn't buy it. The inventor of Ibuprofen's confidence in his kind was surely misplaced. Scientists were only human, and subject to the same pressures as the rest of us – personal, financial, political. Besides, how could anyone possibly foresee all the potential risks of a new agrochemical; and where had the agrochemical revolution got us, anyway?

I was still brooding on it by the time I got back to London, where I found Melissa tranquilly breast-feeding Amelia.

'Perhaps Drummond was applying the therapeutic ratio when he accepted the job,' she said, when I related my conversation with Hobday. 'Maybe he calculated that the potential financial benefits to his family outweighed the potential risk to his scientist's ideals.'

'But that doesn't compute. He was responsible for marketing Dichlorprop, for God's sake. Yet even Hobday said he was an altruist. He can't have been such a hypocrite.'

'Altruists are human too. Maybe he just took his eye off the ball. His research department was doing a lot of other stuff too, wasn't it? Nice, altruistic stuff for the benefit of the Third World. Maybe he just made a mistake with the Dichlorprop.'

'But I still don't get why he went to Boots in the first place. Agrochemical development was one of their core businesses. He must have known what the job would entail. I just don't think he was the kind of man who would sell out like that.'

'Aren't you exaggerating a bit? Here, hold the baby for a minute.'

I cradled Amelia as Melissa buttoned up her shirt. The baby gazed back with contented, sleepy blue eyes. She had lost her newborn floppiness so that it was no longer necessary to support her head with the palm of a hand. However chemically contaminated her diet might have been, it clearly wasn't retarding her growth.

'What if there was some other reason entirely for his going to Boots?' I went on.

'Such as?'

'You know – the old French spy theory thing.'

'I thought you said you thought that was all rubbish, and that the Dominicis were definitely guilty.'

'I think they probably were guilty, but I'm not sure about the other bit.

Drummond could easily have been a spy. You've got to admit that a family camping holiday would make a classic cover. What if he really was on some kind of government mission in 1952, and then randomly murdered? The two things could be entirely unconnected.'

'But he wasn't on a government mission. He was on holiday.'

'Only seemingly.'

'Oh my Lord,' Melissa said. 'Not another wild goose chase. You really can be obsessive – you know that, don't you?'

It wasn't so hard, actually, to see where the secret mission idea had come from. There was much to suggest that the Drummond family's presence at La Grand'Terre on that hot August night was no coincidence. Perhaps the most troubling detail was the position of the Drummond car. Police photographs and sketches of the crime scene showed that the family parked parallel to and about one foot away from the N96, a busy trunk road even at night in those pre-motorway days. It was a curiously bad choice for a family of tourists looking for a peaceful night's sleep under the stars. Some fifty motorists later came forward to report that they had noticed the Hillman, positioned as it was on the apex of a shallow curve in the road so that it was raked by their headlights as they passed by. The Drummonds had ample opportunity to select a better spot. They arrived at La Grand'Terre at dusk, when there was still enough light to see by, and there was plenty of space a little further from the road. Just another 10 or 20 feet would have afforded them the shelter of trees and undergrowth. Drummond was a cultured man, a stalwart of the Nottingham branch of the Wine and Food Society on holiday with his wife and ten-year-old daughter, not some long-distance trucker on his own. He was also an experienced camper who knew and loved the French countryside. He was not the type to make the basic mistake of trying to sleep on the verge of a noisy road.

If, on the other hand, Drummond had parked with the intention of being seen from the road, the location was perfect. The car was parked exactly opposite one of the tombstone-shaped milestones that punctuate the borders of all *routes nationales*. This one, number 32, told drivers that they were at the exact midpoint between the two nearest small towns on the N96: Peyruis, 6 km to the north, and La Brillanne, 6 km to the south. Coincidence, perhaps. But if Drummond had pre-arranged a meeting here, the milestone would certainly have been a useful location-finder for the other party. In fact the more I studied the geography of the crime scene, the more I thought I detected the makings of a rendezvous. This could have been perfectly innocent – a meeting up with friends, for example. Yet no such friends ever came forward, any more than the famous woman in black sighted at Digne was ever identified. And if the rendezvous was so innocent, why the remote location; and why did it have to take place in the middle of the night?

There were other clues that the spot had been pre-chosen. It was even possible that the Drummonds had reconnoitred it earlier in the day. Sébeille's investigators had tried to piece together exactly where the Drummonds had been from the moment they set out from the villa at Villefranche, but large gaps remained in the official account. The family had left the villa just after 6 a.m., which was inexplicably early. The sole purpose of their trip – or so they apparently told the Marrians – was to see the *charlottade* at Digne, which they must have known did not begin until 4 p.m. Villefranche to Digne, a 120 km route they had taken in the opposite direction three days earlier, was at most a three-hour drive, not a ten-hour one. Where were they in the intervening time?

A postman, Francis Perrin, told police that at 11.30 a.m. on 4 August he passed a green Hillman driving very slowly down the steep road that led away from Lurs and the tenth-century monastery on the high Ganagobie Plateau further up. The Hillman had GB plates on the back and three people inside: a man, a woman and a little girl. It sounded like the Drummonds all right. But Perrin's sighting was never corroborated. The police had been inundated with dozens of similar sightings from around the region, most of which turned out to be red herrings. The Hillman was a rare car in 1950s France, but its shape was not dissimilar to a model of Peugeot common at the time, the 203. For a while the public reported seeing Hillmans on almost every street corner. The possibility that a genuine, second British Hillman had been at large in the region could also not be dismissed.

For whatever reason, little importance was attached to Perrin's story at the time, even though to get to Lurs the Drummonds must necessarily have passed La Grand'Terre, a few miles down the hill. Once again, their presence in the locality could have been innocent. Then as now, the Ganagobie monastery was a famous beauty spot marked on all the tourist maps, with outstanding views across the densely wooded hills to the north and the whole of the Durance valley spread out below. Lurs itself was also a tourist attraction, an archetypal medieval hill town that in 1952 was in a state of picturesque semi-dereliction. The family might have gone to either place for a walk, or a picnic – unless tourism was a cover for some hidden Drummond agenda.

During the investigation it was widely assumed that Drummond had never been to the region before 1952, but in fact this was by no means certain. In September of that year, just over a month after the murders, a thirteen-year-old schoolboy called Marshall Hughes was rummaging on a rubbish tip in Long Eaton, south-west of Nottingham, when he made a startling discovery: a pocket diary belonging to Jack Drummond. Apart from one corner of the cover that had been burned, the diary was dry and in good condition, suggesting that it had only recently been discarded.

Marshall immediately recognized the name carefully written on the frontispiece. The Drummond murders were still headline news. He took his prize home to his mother, Ivy. Observing that the diary was not recent, but for the year 1947, Ivy didn't attach much importance to it at first, but the following day she bumped into a local councillor, a W. H. Martin, to whom she mentioned Marshall's curious find. Councillor Martin asked to borrow it. Then the editor of the *Long Eaton Advertiser* got to hear of it and contacted the councillor. A week later, a tantalizing summary of the diary's contents appeared on the *Advertiser*'s front page. Shortly after that, the editor handed the diary to Scotland Yard.

Far from being unimportant, the diary apparently showed that Drummond had been an 'exceedingly frequent' traveller abroad in 1947, in June of which year he had finally taken up his post full-time at Boots. His destinations, the *Advertiser* reported, included the Netherlands, Switzerland – and France. Drummond seems to have been a punctilious diary-keeper. In many instances, according to the report, he had made entries several times a day, logged the names and telephone numbers of many of the people he had met, and noted the times and places that his meetings had taken place. The little book was a potential goldmine of clues. Yet the *Advertiser* seems not to have realized the importance of what they had. In the best traditions of provincial journalism they were frustratingly preoccupied with establishing a local connection. They thought it worth reporting the discovery inside of a local telephone number, Long Eaton 937, even though 'there was neither name nor address attached to it, so that did not lead very far'.

Two years later – that is to say, in August 1954, three months before Gaston's trial – the *Advertiser*'s editor, whose name was Thompson, penned a long article for the *Sunday Empire News* (a Manchester-based paper amalgamated long ago with the *News of the World*) in which he made the sensational claim that the meetings mentioned in the 1947 diary included one at Lurs – although he did not say, or else the diary did not specify, whom Drummond was supposed to have met there. If Thompson was right, this was real news. His revelation became a cornerstone of the secret agent theory advanced by William Reymond forty-three years later.

Very curiously, Commissaire Sébeille failed to follow up the new lead at the time. The diary was not even mentioned in the course of Gaston's trial. To cap it all, the diary subsequently disappeared. Reymond wrote that he had searched for it in Scotland Yard's archives, to no avail. In fact, like the conspiracy theorist that he was, he went so far as to suggest that the diary was the subject of an official cover-up. In truth the diary's disappearance *was* mysterious. The Drummond murder enquiry is still officially open in Britain, where evidence relating to such cases is routinely preserved, not destroyed. Nor was it clear how something as obviously valuable to police investigators as a murder victim's pocket diary had been thrown out in the first place. Had someone really tried to burn the diary? Who and why would someone want to hide the fact that Drummond had been to Lurs before? Was the nature of his business there really so secret?

I decided to conduct my own search for the missing diary. Reymond had looked for it in 1997, before the introduction of the Freedom of Information Act, which theoretically obliged the police to cooperate with requests for information from the public. Moreover, he was French, and I had a friendly contact in Special Branch. If the diary really was still in the possession of Scotland Yard, as Reymond claimed, I quite fancied my chances of finding it. It would be worth the effort if it revealed whom Drummond had known at Lurs.

I rang my contact, who agreed that the diary's disappearance was odd. He said it was possible but not likely that the diary had been 'lost', and agreed to have a word on my behalf with a friend of his, a high-up in the Metropolitan Police's Records Management Branch. At length I heard from a records officer called Maggie Bird, who told me she couldn't find a single reference to it. It wasn't in the Met's property store. Nor was it in the so-called Black Museum, the national repository of sinister murder weapons and hanged criminals' death masks. She eventually discovered something else, though, buried in the overflowing box-files of police correspondence relating to the case. You could tell from the tone of her voice that she was almost as fascinated by the murders as I was.

'Oooh, look at this!' she said suddenly, in the course of our third or fourth telephone conversation. 'It's a postcard. Don't know who it's from; there's no name. It just says, "If the Drummond murders aren't all a communist plot, I'll eat my hat."'

That, unfortunately, was as far as I got in my search. As a last resort I

tried the National Criminal Intelligence Service. It seemed possible that
Scotland Yard had passed or lent the diary to their French counterparts
under the auspices of Interpol, and that a record of such a transaction
might still exist if so – but I drew another blank. The 1947 pocket diary
had vanished as completely as the Hillman shooting brake and the
Drummonds' waxwork heads.

Although Commissaire Sébeille paid little attention to the implications
of Postman Perrin's story or to the alleged contents of the diary, the press
was soon very interested indeed. Speculation was rife in the bars and
hotels of Digne that the diary's unnamed contact was an old priest called
Father Lorenzi, a well-known figure in the community who lived a
secluded life at the Ganagobie monastery. This made a certain amount of
sense if one believed, as many did, that the murders were connected in
some way to the wartime activity of the maquis. A cell of Resistance
fighters had secreted themselves in the impenetrable oak scrub of the
Ganagobie plain in 1944, and Père Lorenzi was understood to have
harboured them often in his eyrie monastery. What was more, Lorenzi
was a good friend of Gaston Dominici, whom he had known for more
than thirty years. Some journalists reported that the monastery had been
a collection point for the Special Operations Executive's covert parachute
supply drops. If this was true – and if Drummond really was in the region
in order to recover stolen SOE parachute gold (or to purloin it for himself,
depending on whose version you preferred) – then Lorenzi would have
been an obvious first point of contact for him.

Scores of journalists trekked up the hill to the monastery to see what
they could winkle out of the old priest. But barring an observation that
the Dominicis were a family of 'model citizens' incapable of such a
vicious crime – hardly an accurate description, given that the Dominicis
themselves admitted failing to assist a dying child – Lorenzi never told
any of them anything. His reticence struck many as suspicious. Some
reckoned that he had taken Gaston's confession and was bound by his
faith to remain silent. Others said his reserve was driven by fear of

Communist or *maquisard* retribution. It was never established whether or not he really had met Drummond. The truth went with him to the grave in 1959.

There were other indications that Drummond had a secret side. It was well known that he had undertaken at least two 'special operations' during the war, the best known of which was his visit to the Nazi-occupied Netherlands in May 1945. The details of that trip were first made public in August 1952 by the *Sunday Express*, who even unearthed a photograph taken on the Dutch border depicting Drummond in military uniform. Was he on another special operation at the time of his death, seven short years after the armistice? The world's press pounced upon the story.

In point of fact, Drummond had long been dogged by rumours that he had some 'unusual' connections. According to Joan Peters, the Food Advice Officer who worked with him at the Ministry of Food, the staff canteen was always full of gossip to that effect. Her glamorous and popular boss was constantly travelling abroad, for one thing, just as he had done before the war. He was particularly peripatetic in 1936 when, between January and May, he visited the Netherlands, Nazi Germany, Austria, Switzerland, Czechoslovakia, Hungary, Poland, Russia and the four Scandinavian countries, all, apparently, in the interests of nutritional research. The trip was funded by the New York-based Rockefeller Foundation, a philanthropic organization that had also paid for his Chair of Biochemistry at UCL. But the Rockefeller Foundation was also often associated with the intelligence community. Their supposedly apolitical credentials were badly damaged in the 1950s when it emerged they had cooperated with the CIA on secret mind-control experiments involving LSD. Whatever the purpose of Drummond's European tour, the network of foreign contacts he had built up over the years must have struck any intelligence service as useful.

In 1939 moreover, in another episode much glossed over in his obituaries, Drummond worked briefly at Porton Down, the government's secret biological weapons research station in Wiltshire, infamous today for its past practice of experimenting on humans. Here he conducted experiments into the fitness for human consumption of food exposed to poison gas. The authorities were so convinced that Hitler would bomb London with toxins that by 1940 they had distributed 38 million gas masks to the public. Drummond's expertise in food canning technology, the first line of defence against food contamination, made him an obvious choice for this highly confidential work. That in itself did not make him a spy, but it did reinforce the impression that his association with the secret side of government was an established one. Drummond could not have worked at Porton Down without first being asked to sign the Official Secrets Act.

Drummond, the man, also seemed to me to match the profile of a spy to an extraordinary degree. His provenance remains mysterious: no birth certificate for him exists in the Family Records Office. He wasn't always known as Jack, or even as Drummond. His father, the major, described himself as a bachelor in his will, which made no mention of any son. Jack's mother, who gave her name in the 1891 census as Gertrude Drummond, was twenty-nine; Jack's name was given as Cecil. It is not known what happened to Gertrude, or if she was married to John, or even if her name was really Gertrude. Drummond was brought up by his aunt, Maria Spinks; by the time of the 1901 census, he gave his name as Jack Cecil Spinks.

As an adopted child he had always lived with a double identity. His illegitimacy was socially embarrassing, so he had to teach himself discretion from an early age. Silvia Austin-Smith described the adult Drummond as 'glamorous', but also as a 'quiet and deeply private man', who never once spoke even to them of his family antecedents. Despite his charm, his courtesy, his approachability and his undoubted passion for nutrition, like a lot of adopted people he remained a bit of a blank slate. I counted two or three adopted people among my friends and had always found them intriguing. Unencumbered by ancestry, they tended to be ambitious, driven, more anxious than average to make their own mark on the world. They were existentialists by necessity, and talented at self-invention.

Drummond was a master of that. He dropped his adopted surname, Spinks, and reverted to the one he was born with at some time in his teens. Nothing I read and no-one I spoke to could ever quite explain why. The public persona he finally settled on was the 'people's scientist'. He became the one and only 'Sir Jack' – a man who refused to be called John, even after he was knighted, and who hated more than anything to be called Cecil. He was loved and trusted by all who came into contact with him. Many people, including his close associate Magnus Pyke, noted his steady and uncomplicated sense of patriotism (which derived, perhaps, from the fact that his adoptive father, his true father and his grandfather had all been professional soldiers, and maybe also from his own brief military career). And yet he amazed his colleagues by swapping academia for the world of commerce and industry in 1946; he abandoned his first wife after years of apparently happy marriage for Anne Wilbraham. He was a paradox: John Le Carré himself couldn't have invented a more likely character for recruitment into the secret services. I had the feeling that no-one, not even those close to him like Silvia Austin-Smith, had ever *really* known him.

Chapter 7
Mission Impossible?

'Early in the 19th century a number of new fruits were introduced.
North Carolina sent the tomato or "love-apple", considered by some
authorities to be violently aphrodisiac. It was grown, at first, more
as a decoration than for eating but by 1880 it was being offered for
sale in most of the fruit markets, although for a time there was a
curious aversion to it on grounds of its unusual colour. The absurd
fallacy that tomatoes cause cancer does not seem to have become
current until about 1900. There is, of course, not the slightest
foundation for this ridiculous belief, which is sometimes met with
even today.'

The Englishman's Food

Of course, none of what I had so far uncovered proved that Drummond
was on a secret mission at the time of his family's murder. But the
persistent stories of stolen parachute gold, Postman Perrin's sighting of
the Hillman on the road up to Lurs, and the rumours surrounding the
reclusive priest, Père Lorenzi, did seem to point to some kind of
connection to the maquis. It seemed worth looking deeper into the
wartime involvement in the region of the Special Operations Executive,
the secretive, London-based body who ran and supplied the French
Resistance. So I asked the undisputed expert, Professor M. R. D. Foot, the
SOE's official historian.

One of his books, published by HM Stationery Office in 1966, contained material so sensitive that its first edition had to be withdrawn and amended on the orders of Churchill himself. Now eighty-six, Foot fought in France with the Royal Artillery and was decorated for his work alongside the Resistance in Brittany in 1945. He was an erect, donnish man who spoke in the unreconstructed tones of his classically educated generation. He spoke almost in note-form when I met him, omitting articles, pronouns and any other grammar that he considered superfluous to his meaning, so that his anecdotes came out in bursts like a gun spitting bullets. He was mesmerizing: I had never heard 'circa' pronounced with two hard *c*s before.

He explained how the SOE had divided German-occupied France into six sections, to which over 1800 secret agents had been deployed in the course of the war. They operated in 'circuits' of various sizes that enjoyed prosaic codenames like 'Ventriloquist', 'Newsagent' and 'Wheelwright'. He remembered the murders of 1952, as people of his age tended to. He had also heard the rumours that Drummond was connected to the SOE. He had never given them much credence, although he didn't rule out the possibility: even he didn't know the names of all 1800 of the agents deployed before 1945. The circuit covering the Basses-Alpes region had been called 'Jockey', which was set up by a Colonel Francis Cammaerts, DSO.

'Very good man, Cammaerts. Half-Belgian. Born: England. School-teacher in Penge. War starts. Registers as conscientious objector. Then brother killed: RAF. Cammaerts changes mind. Joins SOE, circa June '42. Codename "Roger". Joins "Donkeyman", but "Donkeyman" penetrated; so sets up "Jockey". Best circuit in France. Go and ask him about Drummond,' Foot concluded suddenly. 'He lives near Montpellier. I'll warn him you're coming.'

Before Montpellier I returned to the Public Records Office in Kew. Foot had told me how and where to look for information on SOE recruitment, although he also warned that much information had still not been released, even now. The thirty-year rule on disclosure did not always apply where the secret services were concerned. If government mandarins judged that a matter was still too sensitive for public consumption, they were empowered to extend the period of suppression to 40, 75 or even 100 years. I spent a morning sifting through piles of yellowing documents but could find no evidence linking Drummond either to the SOE or to any other secret service, although there was plenty to speculate about in the files. A letter from Grenoble was typical: its author, M. D. Orson, claimed to 'know where the documents that Monsieur Drummond was seeking are to be found'. There was also a Victor Hasenfratz of Digne, who had written to Scotland Yard in 1964, a full decade after the trial, to accuse Gustave Dominici of the murder of an English parachutist during the war and the theft of 7 million francs. This man described Gustave, in throat-clearing patois, as *'un criminel de guerre'*: a war criminal.

I flew to Montpellier by Easyjet and rented a car for the hour's drive to Cammaerts's house. Foot's thumbnail sketch of the colonel's career, I discovered, didn't begin to do justice to the man. By D-Day, less than two years after setting up Jockey, he could call on an armed underground network 15,000 strong. To the French, he was a living legend. In a memoir, an SOE colleague depicted him 'striding across the uplands, his tall figure causing the shepherds to call to each other, *"Voilà le grand diable d'anglais"*; for among the simple, honest people of the region, his nationality could not be hidden. There was not a man among them who would not have fought to save him; not a woman who would not have hidden him from pursuit at the risk of her life; not a child who would not have undergone any form of torture rather than betray *l'ami anglais*.' Dodging the Nazis required an ability to think fast as well as enormous courage. Cammaerts was once stopped at an SS control point at Avignon train station. He bit his lip hard enough to draw blood, coughed and spluttered, and spat red on the platform. The Germans, Cammaerts knew, were terrified of tuberculosis. His papers were returned very quickly and he was sent on his way. He was caught only once and imprisoned briefly by the Germans at Digne – the same prison, coincidentally, in which Gaston Dominici was held nine years later.

The sleepy market town in Hérault where Cammaerts now lived had a pretty church but was otherwise unremarkable. A trio of old men standing by a garden gate, one of them wearing a veteran's beret, seemed to be watching closely as I got out of the car. As I headed towards the Cammaerts house, one of them stepped forward, said *'Bonjour'* and started a long conversation about the weather. They knew who I was on my way to see all right. It was if the war had only just ended.

The former giant of the Resistance had shrunk into a thin and frail old man of 89. He had given strict instructions to come at eleven o'clock because that was when he was at his best; at other times of the day there was a risk that I might find him asleep. His clothes no longer fitted him – the top button of his shirt was done up, but there was still room to fit a hand in the gap between collar and neck – and he spoke in a tremulous whisper that my tape recorder struggled to pick up. Yet despite his weakened state a residual toughness was apparent. He was impatient with my questions about stolen parachute gold and all the other theories about SOE involvement, and snorted sarcastically when I mentioned the letters from M. D. Orson and Victor Hasenfratz, neither of which names meant anything to him.

'Rubbish, it's all rubbish,' he said. 'People have always made the most outrageous claims about the Resistance, particularly people who weren't involved. I assure you there's nothing in it.'

He knew who Drummond was, all right – he even described him as 'the most important civil servant of the war' – but he was equally categorical that Drummond had had nothing to do with the SOE during the war, and that any suggestion to the contrary was just idle chatter. The police had come to ask him the same question in the years after the murders, and he hadn't been able to tell them anything, either. He explained that he had helped to establish the Resistance cell on the Ganagobie plain in 1943, one of about fifty that he assisted in the wider region. The cell's main task was to attack enemy lines of communications: railways, telephones and electricity cables. A hydro-electric station on the Durance, he recalled, was sabotaged.

'It was a relatively small cell with a parachute drop-zone that did receive some materials, but only twice.'

The stories of gold and millions of francs were evidently wildly exaggerated, as was the role of Père Lorenzi. Cammaerts had never heard of him, either. This was disappointing, for I had convinced myself that I was on a hot trail. There was a consolation prize that I had not anticipated, however: Cammaerts had known Gaston Dominici slightly during the war.

The maquis, the old soldier explained, had expected the American-led second front to materialize in 1943, but by October it was clear that the advance from the south would be delayed until the following year. This created a huge logistics problem for the Resistance. Hundreds of young volunteers had joined them in the mountains that summer, bringing no food or proper clothes with them – and it was now winter.

'What could we do? We couldn't send them back to their villages, they'd have been killed. So we asked all the local farmers to hive off part of whatever they produced – not too much, or the Germans would have noticed – and we'd go down to collect it, or else they would bring it up themselves. Gaston Dominici was one of the farmers who agreed to help us. He brought sheep, tomatoes, table-grapes – that sort of thing.'

'And what did you think of him – was he capable of murdering the Drummonds?'

'Of course he was,' said Cammaerts, with a disconcerting gleam in his eye. 'These are rough people you're talking about. I remember the murders well. A close friend of mine, a butcher, lived in the area and knew the Dominicis. He was sure the old man was guilty.'

'But what was the motive?'

'You don't always need a motive to kill people,' he shrugged.

I went back to London and started again. I was not too discouraged.

Drummond's death might have been unconnected to what had gone on in the Durance valley during the war, but my conviction that he had been there in 1952 for a clandestine meeting about something remained unshaken. I began to explore other avenues. The journalist William Reymond's principal theory was that Drummond was assassinated by a KGB hit-squad because he was a British agent working for Operation Paperclip. According to this scenario, Drummond had been double-crossed and the rendezvous was a trap. He had gone to Lurs hoping to collect some sensitive piece of information, or perhaps even a useful Eastern Bloc scientist or two, but the KGB killers had got to him first.

It sounded far-fetched. There was no evidence that Drummond was involved in Operation Paperclip or even its British sub-programme, Operation Matchbox. Furthermore, the suggestion of KGB involvement rested entirely on the testimony of one Wilhelm Bartkowski, who was arrested in Stuttgart five days after the murders on an unrelated burglary charge and who confessed spontaneously to a role in the killings. He told the German police that the crime had been committed by a group of three fellow criminals, a Greek, a Spaniard and a Swiss, who had hired him as their getaway driver. All four men were wanted by German police; Bartkowski said that one of them had carried out 'contract work' for a Communist organization in Frankfurt.

A police investigator from Paris, Charles Gillard, was sent to interview Bartkowski in Stuttgart in November 1952 but quickly dismissed him as a crank. Reymond interviewed him again forty-five years later and declared to the world that, no, Bartkowski's story was certainly true. Then in 2003 Reymond's main rival, the journalist and documentary maker Jean-Charles Deniau, visited the KGB archives in Moscow. He found no record of any assassination mission in 1952, nor any indication that the KGB had even heard of Jack Drummond. Deniau also re-interviewed the self-proclaimed getaway driver in Germany and showed that Gillard had been right all along: Bartkowski's words could not possibly be trusted.

Bartkowski had barely sat down with Deniau before he launched unbidden into a strange yarn about the death of Princess Diana in August 1997 in Paris. He told Deniau that, first, he had been driving in the road-tunnel at the time and had witnessed the famous accident; and second, that the crash was not an accident but a covert assassination ordered by Buckingham Palace. The similarity between the Drummond and Diana incidents was more than obvious. Both contained elements of mystery, both attracted popular conspiracy theory, and both had been massively hyped by the media. (Deniau observed further that both involved the death, in France, in August, of an aristocratic English woman called Lady D, with Bartkowski looking on from behind the wheel of a car.)

Bartkowski had revealed himself to be a sad fantasist, a Walter Mitty-type who liked to imagine himself at the centre of infamous tragedy. Psychiatrists call this relatively common mental illness 'mythomania'. He could not be blamed for his fabrications. If the fault lay anywhere it was with William Reymond, who had become fixated with proving that Gaston and his family were innocent. Reymond may even have believed it. On the other hand he might just have been a clever hack who had got on to a great story, and who wasn't going to let anything like facts get in the way of it. Even Reymond accepted that Gaston's trial was inconclusive. The fact that it was faulty did not necessarily mean that the verdict was wrong. The most that could be said of it was summed up by Jean Giono, the grand old man of letters who covered the trial (and whose birthplace Melissa and I had visited on the day we came across the Drummond grave). 'I'm not saying Gaston wasn't guilty,' he wrote after the trial. 'I'm only saying he was never proven to be so.'

The whodunnit aspect of the murders had always engaged the French the most, but I now saw the question of who pulled the trigger, or triggers, as entirely separate from the more interesting issue of what Drummond was doing at La Grand'Terre in the first place. His rendezvous apparently had nothing to do with the SOE – at least not directly. I was nine-tenths certain it had nothing to do with Operation

Paperclip or the KGB, either. That left a third popular explanation: Drummond was hoping to meet someone who had promised to pass on industrial secrets (with its inevitable corollary: that his contact double-crossed him and killed him instead).

This theory was based on the presence of a chemical plant at Château-Arnoux-Saint-Auban, 12 km up the River Durance from La Grand'Terre, and also on the (wholly unproven) assertion that Drummond's brief work at Porton Down in 1939 had continued during and after the war. All this had been alluded to in my earlier conversation with Ronnie Payne, although he thought a connection with the chemical plant unlikely. Now I wondered if he had been too quick to dismiss the possibility. I discovered that the plant wasn't just any chemical factory, but an ex-military one that specialized in the production of chlorine: the feedstock for much of the pharmaceutical and agrochemical output of Boots.

The plant's origins were interesting. It had been built in a tremendous hurry on military orders from Paris in 1915, in direct response to Fritz Haber's gas attack at Ypres. If the *Boches* were going to lob gas at their troops, the generals reasoned, then France needed some to lob back at them. It went on to become the most important chlorine plant in France. The factory, still producing chlorine today, was converted to civilian use after 1918; but that did not make it less strategically important in 1952, when the Cold War was running at full tilt and the potential applications of chlorine technology, military or civilian, were not yet fully explored.

Britain had been France's staunch ally during the war, and after 1945 the two countries theoretically stood shoulder to shoulder against the new red threat from the East. Innovation in military technology should have been shared: there should have been no need for cross-Channel espionage. In practice, Anglo-French relations had been immensely complicated by the creation of the Iron Curtain. France under the Fourth Republic was a volatile and fractured nation, characterized by weak governments with even weaker leaders who exchanged places with a frequency that was dizzying. Between 1947 and 1958 there were no fewer than twenty-two changes of prime minister. This made it almost impossible for foreign leaders to forge the bonds of trust and friendship that underpin most successful international relations. Paris looked worryingly vulnerable to Russian influence. It was hard for London to decipher what was really going on. France's leadership certainly leaned further to the left than Clement Attlee: President Léon Blum (1946–7) and his successor Vincent Auriol (1947–54) were both members of the orthodox Marxist party, the unsnappily named Section Française de l'International Ouvrière, or French Section of the Workers' International.

No doubt some of the ideologues in Attlee's Labour Party rather liked what they saw across the Channel, but Churchill, the beleaguered defenders of the Right, and the military establishment of the MoD were alarmed. It did not follow at all that France would automatically share its industrial or military secrets with Britain. There seemed a real danger that such secrets could be passed to the Russians instead, particularly if they were harboured in the Basses-Alpes, a region noted for its fervent Communism. The consequences for the West's race for chemical technological supremacy were potentially devastating.

In any case, in the chemical industrial sector – and most of all in the lucrative new sub-sector of agrochemistry – Britain and France were not co-operating but competing. In 1947, America, anxious to halt the westward tide of Communism, launched the European Recovery Program. The brainchild of Secretary of State George Marshall, the ERP was popularly known as the Marshall Plan and is still regarded as the foundation of modern European prosperity. America gambled, perhaps correctly, that rapid economic development would pull France and countries like it back from the brink of Soviet bloc annexation. Between 1947 and 1951 some $13bn, the equivalent of about $100bn today, was poured into the shattered continent. The money was accompanied by an equally extraordinary amount of technical assistance and cooperation.

France's moribund chemical industry was galvanized. Key workers travelled in large numbers to the US to study the latest production techniques, and returned with their heads bursting with fresh ideas. In many cases, French firms were granted the European licence to manufacture the latest American-invented agrochemicals. Britain benefited from the Marshall Plan too, but it stubbornly declined assistance in the sphere of agrochemical manufacture and development. The country was still labouring under the illusion that it was a superpower in 1947. American wealth made Britain feel touchy. In his manifesto, Attlee had appealed directly to the nation's pride in its capacity for innovation. The implication was that Britain's scientists were the world's effortless best who didn't need help, thank you very much, from their American colleagues or from anyone else.

France had no such pride. One of the chief beneficiaries of the transatlantic licencing arrangements on offer was the giant agrochemical concern Rhône-Poulenc, which had once controlled the chlorine plant at Château-Arnoux. Between 1947 and 1955, I discovered with mounting excitement, Rhône-Poulenc manufactured the American-invented, chlorine-based herbicides 2,4-D and 2,4,5-T, the eventual constituents of Agent Orange. They also made a related American herbicide, 2,4-DB and, later, Weedazol and Amid-Thin. All these products were at the cutting edge of agrochemical development, and as such were bound to attract the interest of Whitehall's defence specialists. Some of Rhône-Poulenc's products, very interestingly, were also closely chemically related to the chlorinated herbicides that Boots were developing at the period under Drummond's direction, such as 2,4-DP and MCPP – which was first marketed by Boots in 1953, and so probably in the final stages of development in the year that Drummond was murdered.

Rhône-Poulenc's post-war activities in general were well documented, but information relating specifically to their plant in the Basses-Alpes at the period was curiously scarce. Rhône-Poulenc owned or controlled dozens of chemicals facilities in France, and they manufactured a huge variety of products. Chlorine was a raw material for all sorts of things, notably plastics. It was perfectly possible that the plant did not actually have much to do with agrochemicals. On one obscure website I discovered that there were present-day concerns that the factory had polluted the River Durance with its by-products; in 2000 the local government environmental watchdog, DRIRE, had posted an advisory to anglers to avoid the River Durance around the factory, 'following the precautionary principle'. This was suggestive without proving anything. But then, at the bottom of one of innumerable appendices, I found a short note on remedial action on pollution that had been taken at the plant. 'DEMOLITION OF A FORMER HEXACHLOROCYCLOHEXANE WORKSHOP', it said. 'CURRENT STATUS: WORKS COMPLETED.'

My investigation into the Drummond murders had come full circle.

I rushed downstairs to the garden, where Melissa was weeding, on her knees beside the pram, where the baby slept in the early summer sunshine.

'Oh, hello,' she said drily. 'Nice of you to join us out here.'

'You'll never guess what,' I said.

'What?'

'That chlorine factory. It definitely made agrochemicals.'

'I could do with a drop of weed-killer out here,' she replied. 'Look at this vine thing. It's like a triffid.'

I knew I hadn't paid as much attention to her and Amelia as I perhaps should have done in recent days. I was conscious that I had been more than usually absorbed in my Drummond research – 'Drummonding', as Melissa now sometimes disparagingly called it. Not responding to my latest discovery was her way of telling me off.

'There's something else. The factory used to make Hexachloro-cyclohexane.'

'Hexa-what?'

'HCH. The stuff they made Lindane out of, remember? They only dismantled the workshop a few years ago. Wouldn't it be weird if the factory turned out to be the primary source of the Lindane in our bodies?'

'I suppose it would,' she said, looking at the flowerbed.

'Here, let me help you with that.'

We were silent for a while as we wrestled with the tendrils of the resident *Vitis coignetiae*, a broad-leafed climber so vigorous that it had invaded the next-door garden, prompting our neighbours to complain that it was choking their clematis.

'Your mother called, by the way,' she said eventually. 'She wanted to know if we'd like to borrow their house in France next month, until the end of my maternity leave. It was very nice of her. I said yes.'

'Did you? But that's great! It means I can . . .'

'Yes, I know – finish your Drummond research. But there is one condition. You have to promise you won't disappear on me. You've been so wrapped up in this thing that I've hardly seen you these last few weeks. You need to give it a rest for a bit. I want us to have a holiday in France, OK? God knows I need one.'

'OK,' I said, 'it's a deal.'

Was intelligence-gathering the reason for Drummond's presence in the Basses-Alpes in 1952? He certainly would have been a good choice for such a mission. He didn't need to be working for Porton Down to be qualified: as Boots' Director of Research he knew as much as anybody about the applications of chlorine technology. One of the many intriguing details of the murders was that Drummond's camera, a Kodak Retina 1a that he had brought with him on the trip to Digne, was never found. The explanation most commonly offered was that it was removed from the ransacked Hillman by the Dominicis, because Drummond (or possibly Anne or Elizabeth) had taken an inculpatory photograph of one of them on the evening the family arrived. I found this explanation unlikely. Apart from anything else the Drummonds had reached La Grand'Terre as the light was fading, and the Retina 1a was not equipped with a flash. There must have been some other reason for stealing the camera. Had Drummond perhaps been photographing the chlorine plant?

The opportunity had been there. He and his family had almost certainly passed by the factory on their drive south to Digne on 31 July.

There were also many hours missing from the police account of their movements on the day that they died. Furthermore, Drummond was equipped with the right tool for the job. The Retina 1a looked like a run-of-the-mill tourist camera but it was manufactured by the highly regarded Nagel-Werks factory in Stuttgart and boasted an excellent Zeiss lens. Cameras of this quality were comparatively rare in the West in the 1950s. Drummond, whose passion for photography dated from boyhood, evidently knew what he was doing when it came to selecting his equipment. There was one other detail: Émile Marquet, the traffic policeman on duty in Digne on the evening of the murders, testified that as the Drummonds left the town they stopped to ask him directions not to Nice or Aix or the N96 as might be expected, but very specifically to Château-Arnoux. Why?

In the right hands, I knew, even the simplest photograph could reveal much valuable information about a factory. An enterprising friend of mine, a former army officer who set up a corporate intelligence agency in the 1990s, told me of a job he had once carried out for Enron, the disgraced US energy-trading firm that was bankrupted in 2001. Enron wanted to know how much coal a particular foreign power station was burning, because that would allow them to calculate how much electricity was being generated, which in turn would give them an unrivalled advantage in the lucrative energy futures trading market. My friend's solution was ingenious: masquerading as an ornithologist, he set up a bird-hide, pointed a tripod-mounted camera at the target factory's chimneys, and programmed the camera to take a photograph every hour. The pictures of smoke clouds taken over the following two weeks were passed back for analysis at Enron, who paid my friend £10,000 for his services.

Boots would doubtless have been interested in the goings-on at the chlorine plant, yet I couldn't quite believe that Drummond – altruistic, patriotic, a distinguished senior scientist – would involve himself in something as tawdry as an Enron-style bid for commercial advantage. If he truly was gathering intelligence, it seemed likelier to me that he would have been doing so on behalf of his country. In other words, he was probably working for MI6.

That, it also seemed to me, was the probable explanation for his appointment to the board of Boots in 1946. MI6 has a long tradition of 'placing' its operatives within British industry. The Directorship of Research at a leading international chemicals company was surely a textbook cover-job for an agent. It was the perfect excuse for unusual amounts of foreign travel – at a time when foreign travel was severely restricted – and for asking pertinent questions about chemical technologies that were of specific interest to British national defence. Was Drummond employed by Boots as the result of some discreet conversation in one of the clubs of St James's – the spook-friendly Traveller's, perhaps, or that bastion of High Toryism, the Carlton Club?

Gordon Hobday had told me that Drummond had been 'appointed by the board in the usual way' to his job at Boots, but a corporate history of the company, published in 1974 by the Nottingham University lecturer Stanley Chapman, indicated that the way the board operated was far from 'usual'. Boots' plutocratic chairman, John Boot, Lord Trent, ruled the company as his personal fief, just as his father, Jesse, had done. It was not his custom to consult his board members much. Key decisions, including senior appointments, were often taken unilaterally – a tendency that grew more marked in the years before ill-health forced his retirement in 1953. What or who had prompted him to choose Drummond as his new Director of Research? Lord Trent was a rich and distinguished businessman, but he was also the son of a northern Liberal non-conformist and hardly the Pall Mall type. He was not especially well connected politically, and I could find no evidence that he had any link to the intelligence community.

His second-in-command was a different matter. Educated at Winchester and University College, Oxford, his name was Roundell Cecil Palmer Wolmer, the 3rd Earl of Selborne, and his links to the intelligence community were very strong indeed. More to the point, the deputy chairman was the only member of the Boots board to whom Lord Trent really listened in the post-war years. In fact, according to Stanley Chapman, in his last years the chairman he did little at the company without his Number Two's support. It seemed a racing certainty that this power behind the throne played a big part in Drummond's appointment.

Selborne – 'Top', as his friends called him – was an independent Conservative and, like Drummond's former employer, Lord Woolton, a trusted associate of Churchill. In 1942 Selborne was appointed Minister of Economic Warfare, a large part of whose remit was the running of the Special Operations Executive. He was a noted champion of SOE who frequently used his access to Churchill to secure supplies of arms and planes in the teeth of sceptical opposition from rival government departments. SOE's frontline operatives held him in great affection and knew their supporter at Whitehall by the quasi-codename 'So'. The SOE was wound down after the war, when responsibility for covert operations abroad was passed back to MI6. But personal networks do not simply disintegrate with changes of departmental responsibility; and the interests of capitalist free enterprise (in which Jesse and John Boot were both ardent believers) clearly overlapped with those of the old political and military establishment in the febrile years of the Cold War.

Like Churchill, Woolton and Selborne were both members of the Carlton Club, which, among other things, was a noted gathering place for the right-wing Economic League, a secretive body set up in the 1920s for the upholding of capitalist values and the suppression of Communism. The League was the British version of the 'Un-American Activities Committee' that existed at the period in the US. Its methods were understated compared to those of American McCarthyism, but in the late 1940s it nevertheless actively encouraged captains of industry to vet their staff for political affiliation. Its links to the intelligence services, both formal and informal, dated back many years and were well known in

City circles. It seemed likely that Selborne continued to serve or assist London's intelligence-gatherers after the war. He certainly wanted to. According to his entry in the *Dictionary of National Biography* – revised, I was not entirely surprised to see, by M. R. D. Foot – a proposal of his to use the SOE's worldwide 'friendships' as a base for a permanent peacetime intelligence network was 'brusquely rejected' by Clement Attlee.

There was one other hint that Boots, or Selborne, might have had an interest in concealing the truth of Drummond's connection to the Lurs region. This revolved around the dead man's 1947 pocket diary, and the unresolved matter of how it came to be thrown out. There were really only two places that Drummond would have kept it: in his office at Boots headquarters, or else at his home. If the diary was not kept at the office, then it was removed from Spencer House – which was one of several properties owned by Boots, who routinely offered them as perks to senior employees. The house was cleared out after the Drummonds' deaths, and the paintings and furniture it contained were put up for auction – but not until the middle of October, six weeks after the diary was found. Silvia Austin-Smith thought that one of Anne Drummond's relatives, a sister or cousin, had overseen the depressing business of emptying Spencer House. But that did not alter the fact that Boots held a set of keys to the front door.

If Boots were anxious to scotch the rumour that Drummonds' presence at La Grand'Terre was not coincidental, they were not the only ones. While trawling the police files at the Public Records Office in Kew, I came across an intriguing letter from Guy Marrian, a riposte to an article that had appeared in *Paris Match* magazine in late 1952. The article's author claimed to have spoken to locals who said they saw the Drummonds camping near Lurs on the evening of Thursday 31 July – that is to say, on their way south to the villa at Villefranche. The purpose of Marrian's letter was to emphasize that the Drummonds could not have been camping at Lurs on the Thursday because they had told him they had spent that night at the Grand Hotel at Digne. Given the morass of false information that by this time surrounded the murders, this seemed an oddly small matter for Marrian to single out for correction. It was strange, too, that he had written to the British police rather than to *Paris Match* about the matter. Why was he so eager to dispel the idea that the Drummonds had visited Lurs before the day of their deaths?

Several writers in the past have pointed out the suspicious contradictions in Marrian's testimony before and during the trial. First was his blustering insistence that Drummond was an innocent abroad who couldn't even speak French. In reality Drummond was a talented linguist who spoke it almost fluently, as Marrian must have known. Although he was thirteen years younger than the murdered man, they had been friends for almost thirty years. Drummond had taught him biochemistry in the 1920s at UCL, where he also employed Marrian's wife, Phyllis, as a laboratory assistant. The men shared a love of France. Marrian had first visited the country in 1925 at Drummond's prompting in order to study the effects of vitamin B deficiency.

Second was his explanation for the time the Drummonds apparently took to complete the 117 km drive from Digne to Villefranche on 1 August. The family left the hotel at Digne at 10.30 a.m. but did not arrive at the villa until 5 p.m. Marrian originally told investigators that Drummond had been unable to find the villa, and had spent four hours driving around Villefranche looking for it. Police appealed for anyone who might have seen a lost English car circling the tiny town of Villefranche. Not a single witness came forward. Then at the trial two years later, Marrian changed his story: he now claimed that the Drummonds had filled the intervening time with a side-trip to Aix, an hour or so's drive from Villefranche. No-one ever asked Marrian why he had not told this to the police in the first place. And by 1954 it was too late to find witnesses in Aix who might credibly have corroborated his assertion.

Third, and most revealingly of all, Marrian told Commissaire Sébeille that Drummond had informed him that he and his family would be back at the villa either during the night of 4 August, or else very early on the morning of the 5th. In other words there was something pressing that Drummond had to do before he could return to Villefranche, the precise timing of which was beyond his control: a rendezvous, for example. It seems improbable that he did not offer his old friend an explanation for such strange nocturnal behaviour. Yet within a week Marrian had again changed his story, this time claiming the Drummonds had told him of an intention to camp out on the night of the 4th – even though Marrian's wife told police that she thought this could not have been the case because the Drummonds had deliberately left their tent behind at Villefranche.

All this suggested that Marrian not only knew that his friend was engaged in covert activity of some sort, but also that he had an interest in covering it up. Amazingly he was never challenged on any of his contradictions, either during the trial or subsequently. He died in 1981. But a laborious hunt at the Family Records Office, off Rosebury Avenue, revealed that one of his two daughters, Valerie, was still alive and living at an address in Perthshire. I fired off a letter, jubilant at uncovering the sole survivor of the four last Britons to see the Drummonds alive.

While waiting for a response I found a short biography of Marrian in the library of the Royal Society. He had taught at UCL in the late 1920s before embarking on a distinguished career as a university professor of biochemistry, first at Toronto and then at Edinburgh. He briefly became a chairman of the Society of Chemical Industry after the war, having been elected a fellow of the Royal Society in 1944 – the same year as Drummond – for his pioneer work on the female sex hormone, oestrogen, for which he is still revered by endocrinologists. Yet apart from their time together at UCL, there initially seemed to be no obvious professional link between him and Drummond. His early interest in vitamins and nutrition was quickly supplanted by his specialization in female hormones. The pair were experts in narrow fields of biochemistry that had little to do with each other.

The war years were the link. Like Drummond, I discovered, Marrian was taken off his academic duties in 1939 and seconded to the government – in his case, to the Ministry of Supply. He soon found himself collaborating with scientists from Porton Down on AsH_3, a poison gas called Arsine that Whitehall's intelligence experts then thought the Luftwaffe were most likely to drop on London. At the outbreak of war, therefore, both Drummond and Marrian were specialists in poison gas technology.

Marrian took his new area of expertise a step further than his old mentor. In 1941 he was invited by Canada to join a new chemical warfare field station at Suffield, Alberta. He was released by the Ministry of Supply and went to work there for a year in the summer of 1942. Suffield today is notorious for its wartime practice of conducting experiments on humans. It was the Canadian equivalent of Porton Down. Indeed, Suffield was partly funded by Britain, and was headed by the former Superintendent of Experiments at Porton, a Welshman called Emlyn Llewelyn Davies. The Suffield project enjoyed the specific blessing of Churchill himself.

The advantage of Suffield was its size: 1000 square miles of semi-arid grassland compared to Porton's 7000 acres of Wiltshire downland. Such a big area allowed the scientists to experiment with gas-bombs dropped from planes. Between 1941 and 1945, some 2500 young servicemen volunteered to be the guinea-pigs. Many were badly injured. Some suffered permanent damage to their health. In 2004 one of the volunteers, Bill Tanner, brought a class action against the Canadian government on behalf of 500 veterans and their widows, who were demanding compensation. Interviewed in the *Toronto Globe and Mail*, Tanner recalled being ordered to crawl through a bomb crater filled with mustard gas. He was eighteen at the time, and no-one had warned him what the 'tests' he had volunteered for would entail. 'My hands, arms, neck and forehead were burned into huge, oozing blisters,' he told reporters.

Similar experiments were taking place at Porton. Between 1939 and the 1960s about 20,000 servicemen volunteered to take part in biological and chemical weapons trials. The justification for human experimentation offered by one senior Porton official, quoted in Rob Evans's book *Gassed*, was curiously reminiscent of Gordon Hobday's defence of Thalidomide: 'Experiments with various species of animal to determine the toxicity of chemicals often produced differing results . . . Tests on humans had to be done to discover just how poisonous a compound was to mankind.' In 2002 a new inquest was announced into the death in 1953 of Ronald Maddison, a young RAF mechanic who had been told he was helping research into the common cold. In reality he was subjected to a test involving Sarin, a nerve agent invented by Germany in the 1930s. Maddison's death was finally ruled 'unlawful' by the High Court in London in 2004.

Sarin and mustard gas were just two of dozens of noxious substances experimented upon at Porton and Suffield. After the mustard gas, the Canadian Bill Tanner was exposed to pure chlorine – the original but still one of the most effective poison gasses available to the military in the 1940s. His breathing was so impaired that he was immediately hospitalized; later on he was diagnosed with pneumonia. Not for nothing did the hapless victims of these experiments nickname Suffield 'Sufferville'.

In purely chemical terms the strongest connection between Drummond and Marrian during and after the war was chlorine. Despite three decades of technological progress the element was still the basic building block of most poison gases. Given his experiences in Canada it was hard to believe that Marrian had not been aware of the ex-military facility at Château-Arnoux. And if the plant really was the target of a covert intelligence operation, the villa at Villefranche 70 miles to the south was as good a base as any from which to mount it. To holiday much closer might have looked suspicious. A villa on the Riviera looked more normal, and was close enough not to be too inconvenient.

My excitement at tracing Valerie Marrian was short-lived. She didn't want to meet or even talk. By return of post she said that she had barely known the Drummonds; she had no anecdotal recollections nor anything else that she could possibly contribute. I wrote again – twice – pleading for a short interview, but failed spectacularly to mollify her. Her final reply was typed. My questions, she wrote in best Perthshire English, were 'impertinent'; my theories were 'offensive'. She said she was unaware of her father's wartime work, but that even if she had been she 'certainly would not discuss top secret information'. She ended by saying that she would regard any further approach as harassment.

The exercise wasn't entirely wasted. There were two interesting revelations among her barrage of denials. The first was that, however close Drummond and her parents had been in the 1920s, by 1952 the families were not the 'close friends' that the press once made them out to be. The Marrians had moved to Toronto in 1933, and to Edinburgh after the war, while the Drummonds lived in London and Nottingham. Apart from 'a couple of occasions', the families hadn't seen each other for nearly twenty years. The second revelation was that Marrian had not rented the villa at Villefranche, as the standard accounts of the Dominici Affair all claimed; rather, it was a joint arrangement with Drummond. There was therefore no 'invitation' to France: Drummond was paying for half of it. He might even have chosen the villa. As Valerie wrote, it was a 'rented villa that we [the Marrian family] had never visited before; indeed we had never been in the south of France before, or since'.

I was more convinced than ever that Drummond was on an intelligence-gathering operation in August 1952, and that Marrian was at the very least aware of this, even if he was not an active collaborator. Whatever Drummond's rendezvous had been for, it was evidently important enough for him to wait up half the night at the side of a road. If he was operating under cover of a family holiday, he either tragically underestimated the danger of the meeting he had planned, or else he and his family were the unlucky victims of violence unconnected with his work.

I remembered Silvia Austin-Smith's earlier remark about the normally abstemious Drummond drinking heavily at Spencer House on the eve of his family's departure for France. It made more sense now. I imagined the great nutritionist propped against his drawing room mantelpiece, staring distractedly into a tumbler of whisky as Elizabeth ran about in a state of over-excitement, and Anne worried about what to pack and who was going to feed their daughter's pony while they were away. It was the image of a tired man, neither as young nor as well as he once was, deeply preoccupied by the difficult and possibly dangerous mission that he had been called upon to undertake.

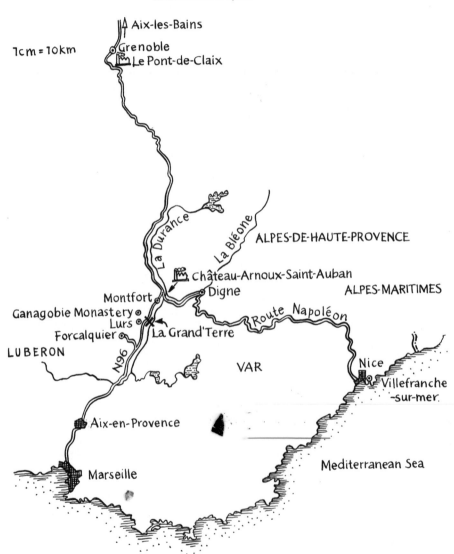

The Basses-Alpes

1cm = 10km

Aix-les-Bains
Grenoble
Le Pont-de-Claix

La Durance

La Bléone

ALPES-DE-HAUTE-PROVENCE

Château-Arnoux-Saint-Auban

Montfort Digne

ALPES-MARITIMES

Ganagobie Monastery
Lurs
Forcalquier La Grand'Terre

Route Napoléon

LUBERON

N96

VAR

Nice
Villefranche
-sur-mer

Aix-en-Provence

Marseille

Mediterranean Sea

Chapter 8

In France

'In the days of good Queen Elizabeth, when mighty Roast Beef was the Englishman's Food, our cookery was plain and simple as our manners; it was not then a science or mistery. But we have of late years refined ourselves out of that simple taste, and conformed our palates to meats and drinks dressed after the French fashion. The natural taste of fish or flesh is become nauseous to our fashionable stomach. All the Earth, from both the poles, the most distant and different climates, must be ransacked for spices, pickles and sauces, not to relish but to disguise our food. This depraved taste of spoiling wholesome dyet, by costly and pernicious sauces and absurd mixtures, does not confine itself to the tables of the great; but the contagion is become epidemical.'

Robert Campbell, *The London Tradesman* (1747),

quoted in *The Englishman's Food*

We spent six weeks in Provence that summer, during which my fascination with the Drummond story did not diminish. I loved the fact that we were a British couple at large in a UK number-plated estate car with our only child, a daughter, in the back. The similarity to the Drummonds' trip to France did not escape either of us. Melissa said it made her feel creepy, but to my mind it was auspicious. Privately, I could hardly wait to retrace their last steps. In line with my agreement with Melissa, however, I put my project to one side when we arrived. Amelia was by now three months old, and we had at last established what approximated to a family routine. She was a sound sleeper, luckily for us, and no longer woke for a feed at three o'clock in the morning. For the first fortnight, and with the house to ourselves, life revolved around the sun-terrace. We commuted from there to the shallow end of the swimming pool, where we swished Amelia through the water until she shrieked with laughter.

The other pleasant preoccupation, of which Drummond would have approved, was eating. Provençal cuisine was one of the main reasons that Melissa was so keen to return to the region. We'd promised ourselves a Michelin-starred restaurant dining experience or three during our stay. By way of anticipation we shopped in the local markets for interesting ingredients with which Melissa experimented in the kitchen. It was possible to visit a different market every day of the week if one wanted, all of them less than 15 miles away. The house was well set up for this activity: every bedside table in the house had a laminated *liste des marchés* pinned to its surface, so that whoever was staying could plan where to shop the following day as they went to sleep. Getting up early was essential if one wanted to catch the best and freshest produce, especially on the fish stalls.

My favourite market was in Pertuis, where the stalls always seemed loaded with the finest of the region. The variety of cheese, wine and olives was reliably astounding, while the fruits and vegetables were of a colour and ripeness seldom seen in England, especially the tomatoes. My favourite was a tiny, sweet-fleshed type of plum tomato known as a pigeon's heart, the skin of which was so red it seemed to glow. Melissa had a chef's eye that was far more attuned than mine to what was special on the stalls. What impressed her most was the seasonality of what was on offer. It was the time for white asparagus when we arrived. Great chunky bundles of it were piled on every stall. They were replaced a fortnight later by yellow courgettes, after which came an equally short Gala melon season, and then juicy white peaches and nectarines.

'Have you ever noticed how you can get purple-sprouting broccoli half the year round in our farmer's market at home?' said Melissa happily. 'That's because they use chillers to extend its shelf-life. None of this stuff has been near a chiller. It's all come straight from the land. You can smell it.'

The head-drilling sunshine, the street-cries of the vendors, and the banter of the *bonnes femmes* as they staggered about beneath their shopping bags added to our sense of intoxication. On the butcher's stands there were cuts and types of meat for sale unknown in Britain, such as udders, or horse. On one occasion we spotted a stuffed pig's nose, and watched as its fat and red-faced vendor explained to a doubtful lady customer that its taste was 'very delicate and subtle'.

'But are you sure it's really clean?' said the lady.

The pink insides of the nostrils gleamed with mucus, and there were course black bristles around their rims.

'Don't worry, I'm always careful to blow its nose first,' the butcher winked, before pretending to blow an enormous raspberry into his cupped hands.

He could have been a character in a novel by Marcel Pagnol. In fact the famous 1986 film versions of Pagnol's 1953 classics, *Jean de Florette* and *Manon des Sources*, starring Gérard Depardieu and Emmanuelle Béart, were shot in several of the villages close by. At night the distant lights of one of them, Cucuron, were visible from the terrace of our house. Small farmers like the pig's nose seller enjoyed an almost mystical status among the French, a nation still in thrall to its vanishing agricultural past. They were seen as the guardians of the idyll of the countryside. In the 1980s and 1990s, when it was fashionable for farmers to block *autoroutes* with their tractors in protest at subsidy cuts, inconvenienced motorists did not complain but raised their fists and beeped their horns in support. This sentimentality explained both the making and the success of *Jean de Florette* and *Manon des Sources*. And it partly explained the continuing fascination with the Dominici Affair, because Gaston was the clog-wearing epitome of the small-holder class, framed and betrayed (if you believed the popular version of what happened) by the evil machinations of the modern state. On the face of things the village markets of the Luberon were a foody tourist's dream: the glory of France and a classic symbol of an apparently immutable way of life.

That summer, however, I was at first unable to look at the markets quite as worshipfully as my family usually did. Perhaps I had been over-sensitized by my research into agrochemicals. An incident early on in our stay certainly didn't help. We had just come back from a shopping excursion in the car. Melissa had put the baby on a rug on the terrace and gone inside for a moment when I noticed that a fine mist was gently raining on Amelia's head. It took several seconds to work out where it was coming from. The garden sprinkler system was off and there wasn't a cloud in the sky. Then I snatched up the baby and hurried inside where I slammed shut every door and window I could find.

Fifty yards up the hill behind the house was an oak-lined vineyard, where a tractor was spraying the grapes. It was one of those specialized tractors with comically close-together wheels that allowed the vehicle to squeeze between the rows of vines. The driver, a walnut-coloured young man in a T-shirt and a broken straw hat, seemed oblivious to the spray drifting down over our house; oblivious also to the risks to his own health, since the tractor cab was of the open kind, and he wore no protective clothing. I never discovered the nature of the substance drizzling from his boom, but whatever it was I was certain it shouldn't be inhaled. For an hour or so afterwards Melissa and I were conscious of a faint but unpleasant tightening in our throats. We saw tractors spraying in other vineyards on two later occasions. These other drivers wore white boiler suits and respirators over their heads that made them look like chemical warfare specialists.

The episode made me wonder how much of the wonderful fruit and vegetables on display in the markets was organic – 'bio', as the French call it – and I soon discovered that almost none of it was. One melon-seller I asked simply laughed and told me I would have to go to a health-food shop if I wanted anything like that.

'Yeah, well,' said Melissa when I reported this exchange to her.

'What do you mean, yeah, well? You're the one who ordered the organic grocery box back at home. Have the rules changed because we're in France?'

'I refuse to live by rules.'

'So all of a sudden it's OK to eat chemical melons.'

'There's nothing wrong with those melons. These people are just small-time farmers. So what if they use a bit of pesticide? It's not as if they're forcing their produce like the big intensive farmers do for the supermarkets – that's the kind of food I really object to.'

'I see! So the goalposts *have* moved.'

'Not at all. It's just that the food on sale here is some of the finest in the world. You can tell that it hasn't been mucked about with. It's all in season and it's all *local*.'

'That's an environmental argument.'

'The environment is important too.'

'Not as important as our health.'

'Darling, you know what? You don't have to eat those melons if you don't want to, but I really don't think they're going to kill us.'

Melissa, it seemed, had already started to think like the French. For all France's love and respect for food, the *bio* movement was a puny fledgling compared to its British equivalent. In 2002 their organic fruit market was worth €54m compared to €330m in Britain (which is still the largest market for organic fruit in Europe). As a nation their view of organic food was at least twenty years behind the British one. Many continued to regard it as the preoccupation of an eccentric and faddish minority. The government was keen on it: in 2001, Paris promised to subsidize farmers who converted to organic production, hoping to double the amount of land dedicated to it to a million hectares by 2005. But the big farmers didn't want to take the risk, and many small-holders were chauvinists who instinctively opposed change. The lure of subsidies wasn't enough, and the government target was missed.

Crop-spray scares aside, it didn't take us long to settle into an easy Provençal routine. Melissa, tired from breast-feeding and the stress of new responsibility, began to unwind as the southern sun worked its magic, and so did I. However exasperated she sometimes was to find me still up after midnight, pouring over Lord Woolton's *Memoirs* or some out-of-print corporate history of Boots – I'd brought a small library of books with me from London – I guessed that she was secretly just as intrigued by the murders as I was. I had gone on about them so much that she had become an expert almost by default. She was an avaricious reader; one day I found her buried in an English-language account of the trial, and when she finished it in a single sitting I knew that she, too, was hooked.

'How about a little Drummonding expedition?' I said later. 'I think it's time we got out of the house.'

'What did you have in mind?'

'I confess I'm looking forward to seeing the chlorine factory.'

'A-ha: Luke Skywalker heads for the Death Star.'

'It isn't far. Forty-five minutes at the most if we take the *autoroute*.'

She agreed, and so the following morning we loaded up the car with Amelia and the baby things and set off up the Durance valley once again.

Heavy industry is not the sort of thing that tourist boards usually promote, so it was a surprise to find a pamphlet about the factory at the visitors' centre at Château-Arnoux. The locals actually seemed very proud of it: the lady behind the desk certainly saw nothing odd about my interest. She explained that some 1200 people still depended on the factory for their livelihoods; 3000, if you counted all those in related service industries. Chlorine was her community's *raison d'être*, just as it had been in Drummond's day. A revealing detail about Jean-Marie Olivier, the ex-maquisard motorcyclist who first brought the news of the murders to the police, was that he was returning home from a night shift at the factory when he was flagged down by Gustave Dominici. I asked if it was possible to visit the plant.

'It's not open to the public,' the tourist officer said, 'but you could always try asking the Director of Communications. I'll give you his phone number. He's a nice man – I'm sure he'll be able to help you.'

The town of Saint-Auban was built next door to medieval Château-Arnoux to house workers when the factory was thrown up in 1915. Nothing had previously existed on the spot apart from the ruins of an old chapel, from which the new town took its name. Saint-Auban gradually expanded to match the original town in size, eventually merging with it to become what the maps now called Château-Arnoux-Saint-Auban or, as the locals sometimes called it, CASA. A village of 600 souls in the mid nineteenth century had become a modern conurbation of 5000, an island of middling prosperity in one of the poorest and most sparsely populated regions in France. According to my pamphlet, the plant had changed ownership seven or eight times over the last ninety years. The present incumbent was Arkema, a subsidiary of the giant petrochemical conglomerate Total, and they produced 145,000 tons of chlorine a year for use in the manufacture of everything from refrigerants and aerosol propellants to PVC floor-coverings, mineral water bottles, shoe-heels and wallpaper paste. Agrochemicals, I noted with quiet satisfaction, were also mentioned.

'In 1915,' I read, 'who would have predicted that chlorine would come to provide the raw material for so many essentials of everyday life?'

The question actually underplayed chlorine's impact on the modern world. Chlorine laid a good claim to be the element of the twentieth century – as important, in its way, as hydrogen and carbon, the constituents of oil. In the global context, the Saint-Auban plant was small fry: the world's chemical industry currently produces an extraordinary 40 million tons of chlorine every year. Since its discovery by the Swedish pharmacist Carl Wilhelm Scheele in 1774 (and its identification as an unusually reactive element by the English chemist Sir Humphrey Davy in

1810), it has proved crucial as an industrial oxidizing agent, for bleaching, and as a germicide. Its contribution to the purification of the world's water supply is incalculable; without chlorine, cholera and many other water-borne diseases would still be rampant. It was central to an agro-chemical revolution that undoubtedly saved millions from starvation in the latter half of the century, whatever view one took of its more recent consequences. It also played a starring role in the post-war plastics revolution that still shapes the modern world. PVC – polyvinyl chloride – is used in far more products than floor-coverings. Plumbing pipes, guttering and other house-building materials all depend on the substance. So do the enclosures for most household electronic equipment such as computers, televisions, hi-fis, even kettles. A PVC variant, polyvinylidene chloride or PVDC, is used in shrink-wrapping and cling-film. Even paper is made from wood-pulp bleached with chlorine. It used to be said in London, rather implausibly, that one was never more than ten feet away from a rat. It is demonstrably true that one is seldom more than ten feet from something containing or depending on chlorine.

The modern world's harnessing of the seventeenth element in the periodic table has come at considerable cost. Organochlorines, of which some 11,000 are currently produced in the world, now dominate every list of hazardous pollutants in existence. Chlorofluorocarbons, still widely used as refrigerants and propellants, are blamed for the depletion of the ozone layer. There was also the small matter of our bodily contamination with Lindane and all the other chlorine-based agrochemicals that our tests had revealed. It is a moot point whether or not Scheele's great discovery was ultimately to the advantage of mankind. As Joe Thornton wrote in *Pandora's Poison*: 'After just six decades of large-scale chlorine chemistry, we can now say that every person and animal on earth is exposed to a complex stew of toxic organochlorines, from the moment of conception – even before, since the developing sperm and egg encounter these poisons too – until the closure of death . . . Even if we stopped all further pollution today, these compounds would remain in the environment, the food web, our tissues and those of future generations for centuries.' I tended to side with Thornton. His book was more credible, at any rate, than the propaganda disseminated by the mighty US-based Chlorine Chemistry Council, whose Old Glorified website was presumably written after the terrorist attacks of 9/11: 'For more than a century, the chemistry of chlorine has helped America to thrive in a changing world. Today more than ever, chlorine keeps America strong and makes our world a safer place.'

There was another pamphlet of interest on display in the tourist office. Among the advertisements for hotels, gliding lessons and canoe hire was a small box of text offering guided walks and, by appointment only, 'Bonsai tree animation'. The name on this strange advertisement was one Claude Dominici. I had never heard of Claude and presumed he must at best be a cousin of the clan, but I noted his telephone number anyway and rang him as soon as we were back in the car. Apart from anything else, Melissa was curious to learn what Bonsai tree animation might entail. She had an irresistible vision of Ken Dodd's Diddymen bouncing up and down in a miniature French forest. In the end we never did find out.

'*Écoutez,*' said the lugubrious voice on the other end. 'It's true that I do Bonsai animations, but only for friends, never for the public. It was just an idea the tourist office had. I didn't know they were going to put it in their pamphlet. I wish they hadn't, to tell the truth. People keep ringing me up. I suppose I might do animations one day but not now. Next year, maybe.'

Claude turned out to be not a cousin but the younger brother of Alain, another son of Gustave. The family had evidently not quit the valley, despite the selling off of La Grand'Terre after the trial and the traumatic associations that the region must have held for them. This was still their *terroir*. Claude revealed that Alain, the leader of the campaign to clear the Dominici name, also lived close by, although he was reluctant at first to tell me precisely where.

'Why do you want to talk to him?' he said when I asked.

'I'm writing about Sir Jack Drummond.'

'Alain gets pestered by journalists all the time,' he said bluntly.

'I'm not a journalist,' I said, 'I'm a historian. *Un Anglais*, from London, writing a book. My main interest is in chemicals and nutrition.'

There was a pause as he processed this.

'OK, I'll speak to him for you. But no promises.'

The directions to the factory given by the lady in the tourist office were clear, but Melissa and I still managed to get lost. Saint-Auban wasn't large, but its streets were confusing. There was no real centre to the town, just a grid of leafy avenues named after forgotten French chemists – Badin, Cordier, Sainte-Claire Deville. The villas set equidistantly along them each had a large square garden attached. These were dotted with children's plastic bric-a-brac, vegetable patches and oil tanks half-hidden by topiary screens. Saint-Auban was completed in 1949, right in the middle of the chlorine boom. It was a model town built for a model workforce that looked more like a transposed piece of mid-American suburbia than Provence.

We saw almost no-one around – the workers were presumably all working – until at the southern edge of town, just before the entrance to an airfield and gliding club, we came across a large encampment of gypsies. At least fifty mobile homes were parked in an untidy circle, in curious contrast to the orderly right-angles of the town we had just driven through. Washing hung on lines strung between the vehicles, each of which was topped by a TV satellite dish trained on the same invisible spot in the cloudless sky. A group of dark brown children stopped their game of football and stared as we approached. We didn't stop to ask for directions.

The factory was to the east of the town and below it, ranged along the alluvial flood plain of the Durance. I felt foolish for not having found it sooner. The place was so colossal that it was impossible to fit it all into the frame of my camera, even from the vantage point of the plateau above. I later learned that it covered 108 acres, a spectacular tangle of silver sheds, steel pipes, railway lines, and red and white chimneys that sprawled like a strange metal vine along the riverbank. An access road wound down the steep escarpment, guarded by a triangular warning sign with the legend 'ATTENTION – SANGLIERS!' beneath the silhouette of a charging wild boar – a reminder that, for all its size, the factory was still no more than an outpost of modernity in the vast bas-alpine wilderness. To the south glinted the spot where the River Bléone joined the Durance, its icy blue waters flowing down from Digne, where Gaston Dominici was put on trial. Giant hills, the foothills of Europe's greatest mountain range, surrounded the confluence on all sides.

This picturesque site had been chosen in 1915 for many reasons. There was an abundant supply of water, essential to the electrolysis process by which chlorine is still produced. It already had good rail-links, and was relatively close to the salt pans of the Camargue, a virtually limitless source of the sodium chloride from which chlorine is extracted. The Mistral wind would blow away any escaped gas in a region that was in any case thinly populated. It was also deemed far enough away from the Western Front to be safe from German attack. Keeping the factory out of sight had evidently not been a criterion, because it was visible for miles in every direction except the west. The need for secrecy would have come later, in the 1940s and 1950s, by which time the world had changed and the factory had diversified from the manufacture of simple chlorine. But in such an exposed location it would have been as easy for Jack Drummond to take photographs then as it was for me now.

I phoned the factory's Director of Communications, a Jean-François Gil, who was unhelpful at first. Arkema used to offer public tours of the plant, he said, but they had been discontinued for the same post 9/11 security reasons given by Boots in Nottingham. I persevered though, and eventually he seemed to relent.

'Write me a detailed letter explaining why you want to come here,' he said. 'I'll show it to my bosses and see if I can make an exception for you. But no promises.'

Melissa and I went back to our holiday. The expedition with the baby to Saint-Auban was such a success that we began to explore further afield, just as we had before we got married. We re-immersed ourselves in France. It turned out to be an interesting time to be there. I had been travelling to the country all my life, yet more than at any time I could remember it seemed to be on the back foot that summer. Contrary to its usual stylish swagger, the place felt somehow ill at ease with itself – uncertain, perhaps, of its direction and place in the world. The contrast with brash Britain had never seemed so great.

The clearest symptom of the malaise came when the public voted to reject a treaty ratifying the new EU constitution, much to the astonishment of President Jacques Chirac, who had blithely described the treaty as a simple 'tidying-up exercise'. The vote was an unprecedented setback for the European project of which France had been the proud motor for more than forty years. Chirac's humiliation was compounded when France lost its bid to host the 2012 Olympics to its oldest sparring partner, Britain. The French sulked like children and accused Tony Blair of underhand lobbying tactics; the British, equally childishly, crowed with undisguised glee.

The constitution's rejection was partly a punishment for the arrogance of Chirac and the political elite in Paris that he represented, but France's middle classes were also genuinely disquieted by the direction of the European project. The newspapers were filled with scare-stories about the effects of EU expansion in eastern Europe. Migrant workers from Poland were undercutting the indigenous construction industry; gypsies from the Czech Republic and elsewhere risked sparking a crime-wave that would inflame the racist right; the entire EU would be overwhelmed. The fear that expansion would somehow lead to a dilution of indigenous culture was hoary in Britain but a relative novelty to France, where Europhobia had suddenly gone mainstream. A shopkeeper told me that he and his wife had voted *non* to the Constitution for the simple reason that they were 'Gauls' – a term that candidly evoked ancient racial rather than modern national solidarity. Gallic xenophobia reached new heights later in the year, when disaffected young Muslims torched thousands of cars in towns across France: the worst urban rioting since 1968.

The politicians in Paris, their confidence already shaken, were mortified to find that the eastern Europeans were in any case not very interested in adopting the French socio-economic model. This seemed the height of ingratitude. Had France not pushed harder and longer than anybody to let them join the EU club in the first place? In the newspapers, bafflement turned to outrage when Tony Blair suggested that the free-market British model might serve the new Europe rather better than the French one. He even had the temerity to suggest that France, too, might benefit from a little deregulation. 'Now Blair wants the Anglo-Saxon model in France!' shrieked a headline in *Le Monde*.

In point of fact, the Anglo-Saxon invasion had already begun. Friends living near Carcassonne reported that the locals were complaining bitterly at rising property prices, and the fact that they could not compete with British buyers who were colonizing the area faster than bees. This was true of the Luberon too, especially the north side of the ridge with its associations with Peter Mayle, the best-selling author of *A Year in Provence*. The nearby town of Apt had a pub called the Queen Vic. Even more symbolic of the perceived assault on French values was a display we spotted in our local *hypermarché* dedicated purely to English cheese. What better illustration could there be of France's unwilling prostration before the forces of global competition? Cheese defined the French. Just before the invasion of Iraq, Matt Groening's cartoon creation Homer Simpson described America's most intransigent European allies as a bunch of 'cheese-eating surrender monkeys' – a description that perversely delighted a Parisian friend of mine who translated it as *singes capitulards, mangeurs du fromage*.

President de Gaulle's famous remark in 1951 that it was 'impossible to bring together a country that has 265 kinds of cheese' was tinged with pride at the anarchic richness of the country he was then hoping to govern. Compared to Britain at the time, he had a point: during the war the Ministry of Food had stipulated that only one type of cheese could be manufactured, a dispiriting-sounding product called 'National Cheese', and it took many years for the industry to recover. By 2005, however, Britain actually had slightly more kinds of cheese than France. Over 400 cheeses were registered with the British Cheese Board compared to the mere 350 or so officially certified across the Channel. De Gaulle would not have been amused.

The Brits have always thumbed their noses at the French, but however sophisticated our national fare might have become, the fact remains that we still eat far less healthily than they do. Just 12 per cent of French people are classified as obese: almost half the British rate and one of the lowest rates in Europe. Their puzzling thinness was a recurrent theme in the women's magazines in 2005, thanks to a book by Mireille Guiliano called *French Women Don't Get Fat*. It headed the *New York Times* best-seller list for months, even though there was nothing new about the Guiliano thesis. Nutritionists observed long ago that the French do indeed manage to stay in better shape than other people, despite the prominence of food and alcohol in their national culture. The anomaly was known as 'the French paradox' even in Drummond's time.

Drummond, of course, would not have used such a word to describe the Gallic physique. The reasons for French good health were abundantly clear to him. As in his day, the typical French meal – a starter, a main dish of meat and vegetables, cheese and fruit to finish – still contains a balance of all the essential nutrients. Nor are the French prone to snacking outside mealtimes as the British and Americans are: they really do just drink café in their cafés.

'Did you know that a third of all the money spent by the British on food is spent on eating out?' said Melissa one day over lunch. As a loyal subscriber to *Restaurant* magazine, she was always reliably full of eating-habit statistics. We were sitting on the sun-dappled terrace of La Fenière, a Michelin-starred restaurant near Lourmarin, where at least two other tables were occupied by parties of British holiday-makers.

'The French don't spend nearly so much,' she went on. 'They generally prefer to stay at home. Everyone knows that traditional eating habits have declined in Britain, but over here three-quarters of all French meals are still eaten *en famille.*'

'I suppose that's good news for British restaurateurs.'

'Not really. The Brits eat out more, but they don't exactly go for quality. Forty per cent of all British restaurant meals involve the consumption of chips.'

We were certainly far from the land of chips here at La Fenière. I had ordered the roast saddle of rabbit in Cucuron olive oil with lemon thyme blinis and aubergine compote, she the fillet of tuna with poutargue, cuttlefish and bacon; and while we were waiting we shared some fried lamb's tongue on a mesclun herb salad with shallots.

Yet despite such culinary miracles and the apparently robust state of the food market at Pertuis, I was beginning to suspect that this Gallic paradise was not all it seemed. Statistically, small farmers like the pig's nose seller were a dying breed. The days of lavish EU subsidies were over: France still received more funding than any other country in Europe under the notorious Common Agricultural Policy, but in contrast to what most people believed, the vast majority of the spoils from Brussels and Strasbourg went to large-scale farmers and rich landowners, not to traditional small-holders. Despite fierce resistance from Paris, France's agricultural subsidy was being whittled away and the funds diverted towards the needier nations of eastern Europe. As a consequence, small French farmers were going out of business at the rate of 30,000 a year. Their numbers had halved since the mid-1980s; they now accounted for less than 4 per cent of the population. The way of life represented by the pig's nose seller was not immutable at all.

Perhaps that explained why some of the markets we frequented felt as though they really only existed for tourists. The Friday market at the *bijou* village of Lourmarin was particularly egregious. It was a theme-park market, a piece of history frozen in garlic-flavoured aspic. The food sellers there were outnumbered three to one by 'artisans' selling absurdly priced bead-ware, yellow tablecloths and pottery decorated with olives, little packets of lavender and suitcase-friendly pots of honey. These artisans were often not locals but down-shifters from the cities seeking their own romanticized slice of the Provençal good life; and the language most commonly heard among the over-paying customers was often not French but English. Lourmarin reminded me of England's Burford, the most chocolate-boxy town in the Cotswolds, where tourists now flock instead of sheep, and shepherds and collies have been replaced by tour guides and coach-drivers.

Even in Pertuis there were signs that tradition was being eroded by market forces.

'Do you see what I see?' said Melissa there one morning, standing by the fish stall, where we were waiting to be served. I stopped playing with Amelia, who was gurgling and windmilling her arms in the sling strapped to my chest. Nestling in the ice among the tuna at the back of the display was a fat slab of Red Label, farmed Scottish salmon.

'*Ahh, il est vraiment très bon, ça,*' said the fishmonger, smacking his lips with the tips of his fingers.

I asked him if he knew where in Scotland it had come from, but he had no idea.

'I just buy it in the fish market in Marseilles.'

We kept an eye out for farmed Scottish salmon in the markets after that, and spotted it almost everywhere. It had been transported across half of Europe, yet it still sold for as little as €12 a kilo, a fraction of the price of local species from the over-fished Mediterranean. *Rascasse*, the pink scorpion fish considered an essential ingredient of the region's speciality, *bouillabaisse*, sometimes cost as much as €39 a kilo.

In Marseilles, *bouillabaisse* had been eaten for so long that it was said to have been served by Venus to her husband, Vulcan, to lull him to sleep while she consorted with Mars. But the final problem faced by the village marketeers was that France as a whole was steadily abandoning the eating patterns of the past. Even if three-quarters of French meals were still taken *en famille*, that still left a quarter of them that were not. The increasing popularity of McDonalds – *MacDos*, as the US chain is known – would have amazed Drummond. At a time of slipping profits in Britain, sales in France grew 42 per cent between 2000 and 2005. Two per cent of the population ate there every day. And although the level of French obesity was half what it was in Britain, it was rising nevertheless. The nation was not really as enviably slim as Mireille Guiliano and others liked to suggest. This was French women's guiltiest secret: in 2004 they spent $230m on anti-cellulite creams and other weight-reducing cosmetics – more than any other European country, and fifteen times more per capita than the Americans.

There was no doubt about it: the modern world was catching up fast with the French. I was reminded of Gaston Dominici in prison in 1954, who cheerily rejected a bowl of tinned soup offered him by a guard with the comment, 'You shouldn't eat preservatives, you know. Preservatives will kill you', before tucking into some bread and home-made sausage instead. The remark seemed strangely prescient – a foreshadowing, perhaps, of the modern organic movement. There was a terrible symbolism in the killing of the famous British promoter of canned food (and harbinger of an uncertain chemical future) at the end of Gaston's scrubby orchard. Drummond had been the big loser in that spectacular clash of cultures, but the tide had turned now. Despite some stout pockets of resistance, at times it seemed to me that the Gaston way of life was crumbling beneath the onslaught of modernity faster than a sandcastle on a beach.

I went to meet Alain Dominici alone. He lived at Montfort, a village just west of Saint-Auban which Melissa and I had noted on our earlier foray. A brooding cluster of ancient dwellings with thick walls and little windows, perched on a conical hill for protection against marauders, it was typical of the region. To motorists passing along the valley below, Montfort's white stonework stood out against the drab mountainside like a mushroom in a field.

Alain was a powerfully built man like his father with large hands and the same handsome, flat face. He spoke French with a strong Provençal twang, although a trace of the old patois remained in his pronunciation of Château-Arnoux as Château-*Arnouks*. On the night of the murders he was allegedly being bottle-fed by his mother. Now he was a school judo-instructor. He lived alone, having moved to Montfort after his divorce ten years previously in a conscious act of self-renewal; he had three children in their thirties who also lived in the region. I was lucky to catch him, he said, because so much of his time these days was taken up by 'judo, judo, always judo'; but since I was writing a whole book on the Dominici Affair and not just a magazine article, I was very welcome.

He ushered me into his sitting room. There were trinkets on doilies, a red leather three-piece suite, and a modern glass-fronted grandfather clock with a massive pendulum wrought in brass. Some of the family photographs on the walls were recognizable from the books he had collaborated on with William Reymond: Alain as a baby in Yvette's arms; Alain as a boy eating fruit with his grandfather looking on. In one corner was the framed Certificate of Merit that had been awarded to Gaston for his role in the apprehension of an armed robber in 1925. The old man used to show this document to visiting journalists in 1952 as evidence of his good character: a Frenchman *'franc z'et loyal'*. Now it was his grandson's turn.

'I swear to you,' said Alain as I peered at it, 'my grandfather never hurt anyone in his life.'

He offered me a coffee, but it was more than an hour before he drew breath to go and make it, and two hours more before I left. The narrative of his grandfather's mistrial began before I had even sat down. Names, dates, times and places poured from him in a remorseless cascade. I thought I knew something about the Dominici Affair, but compared to this man I was a white-belt novice. Like a maths genius with a Rubik's cube, he had picked the details of the affair apart and put them back together again so many times that he could arrive at the solutions he wanted with one arm behind his back.

'I'm still convinced that Bartkowski and his commando were the murderers,' he said. 'There were too many details in his confession that he couldn't possibly have known.'

'What about Jean-Charles Deniau's interview with Bartkowski? Didn't it strike you as . . . peculiar when he started talking about the Princess Diana crash?'

'It's too easy to dismiss Bartkowski as a crazy. Deniau is a jerk: he set out to make a fool of William Reymond purely because William refused to cooperate with him on a documentary he was making. Besides, where's the evidence of what Bartkowski is supposed to have said? Deniau didn't record his interview – and William has Bartkowski on tape.'

He was on firmer ground when it came to demonstrating that his grandfather's trial was a miscarriage of justice. His main complaint was that Commissaire Sébeille, frustrated by his inability to pin the murders on any of the Dominicis and under immense pressure from Paris, had simply invented a narrative that incriminated Gaston and tailored the evidence to fit it. In 1995, Alain said, a dossier had come to light in the archive department at Digne containing potentially crucial material that appeared to have been suppressed at the time of the trial. Among other items it included a blood-soaked shirt belonging to Elizabeth and a second shard of wood from the shattered Rock-Ola carbine. The shirt was found 200 yards from the scene of the crime but not until *after* the famous reconstruction, during which Gaston had gone nowhere near the spot. It therefore cast doubt on the verisimilitude of the entire reconstruction, a central plank in the prosecution case. The shard of wood was equally significant. Gaston always claimed that it was he who found it by Elizabeth's head and handed it to the police, but two gendarmes swore that it was they who had found the shard and that Gaston was a liar. In court, Sébeille advanced this as evidence that Gaston had been attempting to throw his investigators off the trail by appearing anxious to help. The inconvenient existence of a second shard was never mentioned.

There was much, much more – and the longer Alain talked, the harder it became to argue with his quest for a judicial revision. His conviction was total and he seemed to have answers for everything.

'What about the forensic tests on the gun?' I asked. 'Wasn't it proven at the trial that it had been greased with olive oil from Clovis's house?'

'*Ah, non!*' said Alain. 'What the expert said – his name is Olivier, I know him well. He's still alive, lives at Saint-Giniez – what the expert said was that the oil was *analogous* to Clovis's olive oil. He was referring to a similarity at the molecular level, but Olivier wasn't asked to explain himself, and so the court never properly understood. The fact is that the Rock-Ola was greased with a type of mineral oil used by gunsmiths. It hadn't been near any olive oil, which is corrosive and tends to leave telltale marks on the gun-metal.'

'What about your cousin, Roger Perrin?' I tried again. 'Surely you agree that his testimony during the trial was at least suspicious?'

'Ohhh, Roger,' he replied, rolling his eyes. 'The key to Roger is his upbringing. His parents never liked him and his sister was burned to death when he was four. And the trauma . . . *burned* to death, you understand? Consequently, Roger's personality became very . . . agitated.'

'Did he always lie?'

'Roger? *Ooh-là-là* . . . but it wasn't just that he lied. He was really scatter-brained. My grandfather once sent him out for water and he tried to fetch it in a basket.'

Alain was as convinced as I was that the Drummonds had parked at La Grand'Terre for a rendezvous. He also believed that it was the chlorine secrets of Saint-Auban that had drawn Drummond to the region in the first place. He knew a good deal about the factory. Several Dominici relatives had worked there since the war, and before he moved to Montfort he had lived in Château-Arnoux.

'A few years ago I was thinking of writing a history of the factory. I've got a big collection of photographs. Wait, I'll show you.'

The outsized grandfather clock ticked hypnotically in the silence as he went out and returned with a large album. The pages were filled with faded postcards of Saint-Auban, chronologically arranged all the way back to 1915. Flicking forwards through the album as the factory expanded over the years was like looking at one of those time-lapsed nature films of a blossoming flower. In the early 1950s, Alain explained, the factory had begun to specialize in the manufacture of monochloracetic acid.

'AMCA, they called it. It was used to make all sorts of things.'

'Such as agrochemicals with potential military applications.'

'Certainly.'

'And they made Lindane too, didn't they?'

'They did. Lindane was important.'

He thought that Drummond's principal contact must have been a local, probably a factory employee. The mysterious English couple to whom Émile Marquet had spoken in Digne, he believed, were undoubtedly connected to Drummond's true business in the region, although whether the pair were friendly associates or deadly rivals he was unable to say. He claimed that certain 'documents' had been recovered by the gendarmerie from the Drummonds' ransacked car. As soon as the British consulate in Marseille found out about these, a courier was dispatched to Digne to collect them. Alain knew this because he had spoken to the courier himself. From Marseille the documents were sent to London on a special flight, never to be seen again.

'If we knew who Drummond was planning to meet then the mystery would be solved. They're the ones who trapped him.'

'What about the hypothesis that a second Hillman was involved? That might fit with your theory of an English connection.'

'It's possible. William and I asked a garage in Nice that specialized in English cars. They told us there was another Hillman in the region at the time – a white one. The police checked all the Channel ferry ports and found no record of it, but that was because its English owner lived here in France. His name was . . . oh, it will come back to me.'

'Could Père Lorenzi have set up a meeting for Drummond with someone from the factory?'

'I don't think he was involved. What makes you say that?'

'Because Lorenzi helped the maquis on the mountain. They say he had a radio hidden in his monastery for contacting London.'

'Yes.'

'And many of the workers at the factory were ex-maquis.'

'Yes. So what?'

'So if you were an Englishman looking for a contact within the factory – on behalf of MI6, say – and your boss in Nottingham just happened to be the ex-head of the SOE, then Lorenzi might have been a good place to start.'

'I didn't know that Drummond's boss was the ex-head of the SOE.'

'He was called Earl Selborne.'

'That's very clever,' Alain grinned. 'Actually it is even more complicated. The maquis was split into three factions, although around here they mainly fought for the Communists, the Francs-Tireurs et Partisans. De Gaulle was very frightened of the FTP.'

'The British didn't exactly trust the Communists, either. At least, not after the war. Do you think Drummond picked a contact from the wrong faction?'

'It's possible. Or maybe he was double-crossed. I need to give it some more thought. To be honest I never thought of a maquis connection in that way before.'

'I spoke to Francis Cammaerts earlier this year. He was very insistent that there was no maquis connection to the Dominici Affair. The more interesting connection is the post-war one in London between the SOE and MI6.'

'You spoke to *who*—?' said Alain, visibly startled.

'Francis Cammaerts. A great war hero. He was the main maquis organizer in this region.'

'I know who Cammaerts is. Anglo-Belgian. Used to live in the Drôme. Locked up by the Nazis in Digne. William and I tried for months to get hold of him but we couldn't find him.'

'Well, he lives in Hérault now, near Montpellier.'

'But . . . *he*'s the man whose name I couldn't remember just now – the owner of the white Hillman!'

It was my turn to be bewildered.

'Cammaerts drove a Hillman?'

'He did. For my money, he's the missing link in this affair. *He* could have been Drummond's contact.'

'But Cammaerts told me he never met Drummond.'

'Oh, yes?'

'Do you think he was lying?'

But Alain was no longer listening: my talk of Cammaerts and the SOE had set his Rubik's cube mind spinning again. I wondered at him, and the speed and ease with which our conversation had just switched from the far more promising chlorine factory trail. The possibility that Cammaerts drove a Hillman in the early 1950s was not a lead, and to think otherwise was mad. The information was surely irrelevant and coincidental even if it was correct. Cammaerts's Hillman was supposed to have been white; the Drummonds' was olive green. It proved nothing and explained nothing, except perhaps the confusing number of Hillman sightings reported by the public in the aftermath of the murders; unless of course those sightings had been of a white or green Peugeot 203.

Cammaerts was no liar. If he told me he never met Drummond and that Drummond had no connection with the SOE, then that was surely true. If Cammaerts was the missing link, it meant that a decorated Resistance leader was implicated in the assassination of a revered, knighted British nutritionist, his innocent wife and ten-year-old daughter, seven years after the Liberation; and also that he had concealed that link from the French police for more than fifty years. It was too much. Alain was grasping at straws. He had spent his entire adult life in contemplation of the crime, thirty years or more, yet that wasn't long enough. He was still finding new avenues to explore, untested permutations and fresh interpretations of the facts, and would probably still be finding them thirty years from now. I felt nothing but sympathy for him. As Melissa had pointed out, I was prone to the habit myself – and I had only been on the case for a year. The awful futility of his quest, and perhaps of mine too, was laid bare.

Before I left I produced copies of the books he had co-authored with William Reymond. 'To James Fergusson', he wrote on the flyleaf of one of them, the capitals ornate and curly in the old-fashioned French way. '*Avec tout le courage pour retrouver la verité.*' Out in the empty street I looked again at the magnificent view that he lived with. Cars moved like insects along the fateful N96. Down the valley to the left was the edge of Saint-Auban, gateway to the factory of secrets. Somewhere to the right was La Grand'Terre, scene of the family's humiliation and France's shame. It was not a place to live for a man who wished to put the past behind him. Jean Laborde's remark of half a century ago came back to me: '*Pour quiconque s'en occupe, l'affaire Dominici se transforme en obsession.*' It was not a glib observation, I understood now, but the grimmest kind of warning.

Chapter 9

The Factory

'La destinée des nations dépend de la manière dont elles se
nourrissent.'

('The destiny of nations depends on how they feed themselves.')

Jean-Anthelme Brillat-Savarin, *La Physiologie du Goût* (1825),

Frontispiece to *The Englishman's Food*

It took a fortnight of letters and phone calls to get me through the factory
doors. The breakthrough came when I realized that the Director of
Communications, Jean-François Gil, was intensely proud of the factory's
past. His brother and father had worked there before him. He himself had
started work there at sixteen and had never left. He was also responsible
for a recent company history that he later posted me a copy of, *Saint-
Auban – From One Century to Another*.

I presented myself at the guardhouse door on the appointed day and
was shown into a glass box for an obligatory video presentation. Arkema,
I learned, employed 20,000 people at ninety sites around the world, with
a turnover of €5bn. The Saint-Auban plant specialized in the production
of PVC, chlorinated solvents and (as it had done for more than fifty years)
AMCA – monochloracetic acid. The factory's product line had changed
constantly over the years, adapting to market demand in order to survive.
The only thing that had never changed was the base product, chlorine. I
could smell it even in this video room, a thin, acrid, slightly menacing
top-note in the air. Much of the video presentation was about safety

procedure. All vehicles had to be reverse-parked, with the keys left in the ignition; all personnel had to wear goggles and to carry emergency breathing apparatus at all times; all visitors had to know where the emergency showers were located in the event of an accident.

Outside, Jean-François was already waiting. He was a tanned and fit-looking man in his mid-forties who wore a tight black T-shirt and sunglasses propped in his cropped grey hair. We set off on a tour of the plant in his car. The main access road had been dug into the ground under a railway track, deep enough to allow trucks to pass beneath.

'We call this "*la tranchée*" – the trench,' Jean-François said, stopping the car as the road bottomed out. 'In 1926 a chlorine holding-tank exploded and twenty-two people died on this spot as they tried to run away. Chlorine is heavier than air and collected here, you see?'

It was a sweltering summer's day, and the air that blew through the open car windows was thick with heat and the smell of swimming-pools. The significance of the access road's nickname was not lost on me. I had been brought up on Wilfred Owen's 'Dulce et Decorum Est', the war poem that spoke of 'an ecstasy of fumbling' as Owen put his gasmask on, and the 'froth-corrupted lungs' of his poor comrade who wasn't quick enough. It was a timely reminder that this factory, France's first and most important producer of chlorine, was also one of the progenitors of all modern chemical warfare. Arkema hadn't just been ticking boxes with their safety video. I found myself looking more carefully at the mandatory breathing apparatus on my lap.

'Don't worry,' Jean-François laughed, reading my thoughts. 'There hasn't been an incident in at least five years.'

Saint-Auban accepted its first order for liquefied chlorine, 500 tons of it, in January 1916, and was soon shipping prodigious quantities to the Western Front. Chlorine was only the start. Like everyone else, the French worked furiously to improve on Fritz Haber's original battlefield formulation. The new compounds, mostly forgotten now, carried names like Sulvanite, Surpalite and Sternite. Saint-Auban manufactured them all. The most insidious substance was Carbonyl Chloride, better known as Phosgene, the symptoms of poisoning by which sometimes did not appear for seventy-two hours. Victims invariably ended up dead as the membranes of their lungs slowly dissolved. Dichlorodiethyl sulphide, a blistering agent developed late in the war, was officially christened 'Yperite' after the battlefield where gas was first used, although the troops called it mustard gas because of its distinctive colour. There were also some intriguing offshoots of the new technology, such as smoke bombs. One early smoking agent, the French-invented $Zn+CCl(4)+NaClO_3+NH(4)Cl+MgCO_3$, was nicknamed *mélange de berger*, or shepherd's mix, a name that sounded more suited to the shelves of an Edwardian sweetshop than to the murderous fields of Flanders.

It was as well that the Great War ended when it did. By 1918 an estimated 100,000 tons of gas had been deployed on all sides, and fully a quarter of the millions of tons of munitions stockpiled across Europe, Russia and America contained poisonous gas. Both sides had planned an escalation of gas warfare for 1919, when they hoped to insert poison gases into half of all manufactured shells. As it was, some 860,000 people were killed or injured by the new weaponry between 1915 and 1918. The British suffered 188,000 casualties, the French a similar number. Among the French was Jean Giono, who was gassed so badly at Mont Kemmel in 1918 that his eyebrows and eyelids were burned off. Giono was born 30 miles away at Manosque – the same town, coincidentally, as Jean-François – and spent his life in lyrical celebration of the region in which he lived. It would have been interesting to hear his views on the factory, which was both a blemish on his beloved landscape and the instrument of his revenge on the Boches.

Beyond the *tranchée* lay another world. The jumble of pipes, gantries, valves and dials looked gargantuan from this close. The complexity of it all was unnerving and reassuring at the same time. It was like looking at the flight deck of a passenger jet: the overall purpose of the machine was clear enough, yet the details of its operation were incomprehensible. Men in goggles and blue overalls marched about, waving cheerily at Jean-François as we crawled by in the car. The air trembled with the hum of furnaces, electrolysers, compressors and extractor fans, adding to the atmosphere of efficient and ceaseless industry.

There was much in Jean-François's explanation of how it all worked that I did not catch. Some of the language was too technical for me: I didn't know the difference between a chlorate and a chloride in English, let alone in French. He offered no concessions in the speed with which he spoke, and his Provençal accent was thick. Yet there was no mistaking the gist of his words. In his eyes the factory was an extraordinary place, a piece of living industrial heritage.

'*Vous voyez ça?*' he said, pointing at a utilitarian brick and timber workshop. 'It's one of the originals from 1915, and still in use. It was well built, even though they put it up so fast, you see?'

I did see: in places the mortar that held the bricks together splurged out like cream from a squashed cake, and had been allowed to set like that by the time-pressed brick-layers.

His pride was tempered by a certain sadness, however, because all was not well at Saint-Auban. Many of the workshop walls were daubed with graffiti against Arkema's parent company, Total.

'They're rationalizing their chloro-chemicals division,' Jean-François explained. 'This is only one of three factories in the world specializing in AMCA, yet they want to stop production. They're cutting 400 jobs here: a third of the workforce. A lot of people are furious about it.'

The graffiti was certainly passionate. Much of it was obscene. Even the *grands bureaux*, the management headquarters at the centre of the plant, had not escaped the spray cans. '*Total tue nos emplois,*' I read – 'Total is killing our jobs' – and '*Total dans le cul*' (a pithy Gallicism helpfully elucidated by the crudest kind of graphics). More poignant was the wishful '*Vivre travailler, mourir ici*' – 'Live to work and die here' – which suggested a degree of sorrow and anger not seen in an industrial dispute in Britain since Arthur Scargill and the miners' strike a quarter of a century ago. Many local families had served the factory for four generations. The sense of community they felt, Jean-François went on, had not much diminished since the late 1940s and early 1950s: precisely the period of the factory's history that I was most interested in.

Jean-François described Saint-Auban's post-war period as its golden age. Péchiney, the company that then owned the plant, introduced a system known as *'paternalisme'*, by which they effectively bought the loyalty of their workers with a new town for them to live in. Saint-Auban's residents paid no rent for their high-quality housing, and schools and utilities were free; they were even given the first public swimming-pool in the whole of the Basses-Alpes. In 1948 the town became a parish in its own right, separate from Château-Arnoux. The importance of the factory to the nation was confirmed in that year with an official visit by General de Gaulle. The present-day workers had not forgotten the civic pride of those happy times.

It sounded like industrial arcadia, but in reality the post-war period was a turbulent one for the business. Its remote location, an advantage in 1915, had become a handicap in the new competitive environment, and Péchiney were forced into a programme of rationalization. Between 1948 and 1952 some 200 jobs were cut, and output was frantically diversified. AMCA was one of the period's most important new lines. It had many industrial uses, although the one that interested me most was its role in the synthesis of herbicides. In the year of the murders, the factory was busily adding a third AMCA unit. By 1953, the factory had turned the corner. The decision to diversify production had saved it.

Saint-Auban had been involved in the production of agrochemicals since at least 1927, when the first workshop dedicated to their manufacture was built. The pre-war products were mostly simple copper-based formulations intended for use against mildew in the nation's vineyards. It was not until after the war that agrochemical production really took off.

'Sodium chlorate weed-killer was a big deal after the war,' Jean-François said. 'Sometimes it was mixed with other herbicides like 2,4-D to make it more potent.'

My ears pricked up at this: 2,4-D was one of the selective herbicides manufactured by Boots' rival, Rhône-Poulenc, and a close chemical cousin of the herbicides that Drummond's research department was involved with, 2,4-DP and MCPP. The business relationship between Rhône-Poulenc and Péchiney, Jean-François explained, had been close. Rhône-Poulenc were minority shareholders in Péchiney, who supplied them with feedstock and chemical intermediates; they later increased their shareholding and eventually took over the factory.

The other prong of Saint-Auban's post-war agrochemical production drive was organochlorine pesticides. The most significant of these, Jean-François said – just as I had hoped and suspected – was *'Lash-say-ash'*: HCH, the chemical basis of Lindane. HCH production began in 1947. To begin with the gamma isomer of HCH, Lindane, was not extracted on the premises but at another plant at Le Pont-de-Claix, 75 miles to the north – which was owned by Rhône-Poulenc. In 1952, however, Péchiney decided to cut out the middleman by opening its own Lindane extraction unit – the workers called it *'Gamma Pur'* – while simultaneously doubling their output of HCH. Saint-Auban manufactured Lindane from then until 1969, when Rhône-Poulenc took over Péchiney and, presumably for reasons of rationalization, promptly closed the Saint-Auban Lindane unit down again. HCH production was uninterrupted, however. Between 1947 and 1989 Saint-Auban produced 100,000 tons of the stuff, while their chief client, the Rhône-Poulenc plant at Le Pont-de-Claix, went on to become the largest Lindane producer in the world.

Jean-François had a ready explanation for his extensive knowledge about Lindane: his brother had once worked on the HCH production line. The HCH workshop had only been demolished in 1996. The space it once occupied, about half the size of a football pitch, was now an underused staff car park hemmed in on all sides by sheds and machinery.

Jean-François stopped the car in the centre of this agrochemical ground zero and switched off the ignition. The only movement visible was the air shimmering above the baking asphalt. I squinted through the windscreen, wondering if this could be the primary source of my contamination on a Hertfordshire farm in 1984. If so, the Lindane in my body had come home.

'My brother didn't like it here much,' Jean-François said. 'It was a very hard place to work, particularly in hot weather . . . He used to complain that his hands stank of HCH, even after showering. He could never shift that smell.'

The former workshop was never popular with the workers, who nicknamed it *'le bagne'*, the penal colony. The smell was bad enough, but the din made by the unit's air compressors was 'infernal, almost unbearable'. Later, in the corporate history Jean-François had given me, I found an interview with a retired fireman called Robert Tarditi, who had spent almost thirty years with the company. He had travelled all over France to learn different chemical fire-fighting techniques. Chlorine, he told his interviewer, was dangerous enough – he had once accidentally inhaled a small amount of it – but it didn't come close to HCH, which was by far the worst product he ever had to deal with. 'I was frightened of that one,' he said. 'It was really a vile product.'

'Didn't it worry your brother when Lindane was banned?' I asked. 'Because they'd discovered it might be . . . carcinogenic?'

I struggled to find the right French word for this – it seemed not to be *carcinogénique* – until Jean-François intervened, politely enunciating the correct one back at me: *can-cé-ri-gène*.

'He didn't worry,' he answered eventually, 'because he was always careful. He handled all chemicals with respect.'

It was clear that not everyone was so cautious, however.

'Lindane was very powerful. Some of the workers used to take little bits of it home to use in their gardens and if they didn't mix it right it would burn the plants.'

'But wasn't their health affected? For instance, is the percentage of cancer cases higher than average among your workers?'

My guide pursed his lips and was silent for a moment. He didn't like it when our talk strayed towards anything controversial or negative about the factory that had employed him for two-thirds of his life.

'The hospital here has collated figures but only in the last five years or so,' he replied at last. 'There's no evidence of any ill-effects.'

I privately doubted that this was the whole story. I knew from experience how difficult it was to prove a link between chemicals and ill-health. The word 'evidence' was a weasel-word much favoured by apologists for industrial chemistry. Moreover, I had previously put a similar question to Alain Dominici, whose answer sounded more candid.

'People who work at the factory tend to die sooner and more frequently than those who don't,' he said. 'I had an uncle who worked in the carbide unit. They did an autopsy when he died and found he had no lungs left.'

The environmental impact of the factory was another thorny topic for Jean-François. It pained him to admit that some 27 kilos of mercury, a by-product of the chlorine electrolysis process, were found in the Durance each year. At the same time he was adamant that the DRIRE advisory to anglers to avoid eating fish from the river around Saint-Auban was over the top.

'Twenty-seven kilos of mercury is hardly anything,' he insisted. 'It would barely fill a bottle. We minimize our waste. Half the new invest-ment on this plant each year is spent on protecting the environment. A half! It's mad! Compare us to France's dentists, who throw away between 400 and 800 *tons* of mercury every year . . . They tell you it is different because their waste is incinerated. But how is that different? It just goes into the air for the little birdies to breathe. Not very nice, that. And besides, fish caught in the Durance are supposed to be thrown back in. There have been no trout in the Durance for years, only barbel. People don't eat barbel much, and even if they did they would have to eat 300 grams three times a day before there was any risk of poisoning.'

I smiled inwardly. This was the same old argument used by Billingsgate fishmongers in defence of farmed Scottish salmon, by the Food Standards Agency in defence of Sudan 1, even by the US government in defence of Aminotriazole-laced cranberries back in 1959. Whatever the truth, there was no denying that industrialization had drastically altered the Durance valley – and I felt certain that this alteration was for the worse.

The river, dammed in 1962 just upstream of Château-Arnoux, was a trickle of its former self. Only the impressive width of the flood plain beyond its banks gave any hint of its old power. In places the alluvium deposited over millennia had been baked white by the sun, and shimmered like the Sahara. Meanwhile, thanks to the construction of an *autoroute*, the A51, traffic now flowed in place of water. Sandwiched between the river and the old N96 that it was designed to relieve, and opened in 1986, the A51 led north to the Alps and south to a futuristic collision of motorway junctions in the Bouches-du-Rhône. The first fast road-link between the region and the rest of France, the A51, was intended to help the local economy, although to traditionalists it was just one more example of the encroachment of the over-developing world. Jean Giono had once fished for trout in the Durance. He held strong views on its culinary preparation: 'Never with butter, never with almonds,' he wrote, 'that is not cooking, it is packaging.' But, cooked or packaged, the trout had all gone now, just as surely as the slower, simpler life that he had once championed.

The factory made an apt new focal point for this desecrated valley. Never mind the fish: as one of the largest chlorine manufacturers in Europe, Saint-Auban had in all likelihood contributed to the agro-chemical contamination of me and my family. And it was a certain contributor to the chlorine-based pollution of the world in general over the last hundred years. The local tourist authorities could have closed the place down, clapped a preservation order on it, and charged an entrance fee: the plant already felt a bit like a theme park, or else a vast, avant-garde monument to the dangers of twentieth-century industrial development.

I didn't need to prompt my guide to talk about the Dominici Affair. As a local man he knew all about it.

'My father fought for the FTP,' he said. 'He knew Gaston Dominici. He wasn't sure if Gaston was the murderer, but he used to say that even if Gaston wasn't guilty he certainly knew who was, but was too scared to tell.'

'What did your father think was the motive?'

'Something to do with stolen Allied gold. Drummond was taken for an agent from London looking to recover it, and killed because of that. It wasn't the maquis, though. The maquis would never have killed an Englishman. The killers probably had maquis connections but they were really just criminals.'

It was interesting to hear this old suspicion at first hand. The dark undercurrents that swirled through the valley in the 1940s and 1950s were evidently still strong. The war memorial at Château-Arnoux was as carefully tended as any in France. It was also unusually grandiose, a large obelisk studded with the names of *'les morts de la guerre 1939–45 et de la Résistance'*. Around here, that *'et'* suggested, dying for the Resistance was seen as something entirely separate from dying in the war. It certainly still meant something to Jean-François that his father had fought for the maquis. I suspected that it also meant something to him that I was from Britain, the country that had supplied and supported the Resistance. There was a solicitous quality to the way he led me around the plant that I couldn't quite fathom – something more than innate politeness or kindness. Of course it made a difference that I spoke his language, more or less, but I couldn't help wondering if he would have been so willing to bend the visitor rules for a German or even an American.

He was also proud of the factory's resistance to the Nazi occupation. The Germans had kept it running and switched the focus of production to aluminium, a material crucial to the manufacture of aircraft. This didn't stop management from hiding the racial identity of sixty Jewish employees. The workers consistently sabotaged their unwilling war effort, either through covert go-slows or else by secretly co-operating with maquis marauders. It was odd that Francis Cammaerts hadn't mentioned it, but in January 1944 a maquis unit broke into the main aluminium machine hall and damaged it with plastic explosives. Seven months later the factory was completely shut down by simultaneous attacks on a new chlorine unit, the magnesium machine hall and the main power supply. There was a further attack at the end of 1944.

The fighters who came down from the hills at the end of the war swapped their sten-guns for jobs at the factory, but they and the workers who had remained behind were all brothers-in-arms. The Communist ideals that had sustained the maquis in the mountains were seamlessly transferred onto the factory shop-floor. For years in the local consciousness, Communism and heroism remained intertwined. It was no accident that the town war memorial was overtly Stalinist in style. The obelisk was flanked by the statue of a teenage boy standing over a plough, the symbol of peace, with his chest heroically squared and one finger pointing resolutely at the long list of the dead; behind him stood his mother, demure in a long skirt and hair tied in a neat bun, weeping bravely into her hands. *L'URSS* really did once *domine ici*.

The tradition of resistance was still evident in the fury of the anti-Total graffiti on the factory walls. How much stronger must it have been in the period after the war? In the 1950s the new worker town of Saint-Auban was privately owned by Péchiney, beyond the jurisdiction even of the gendarmerie. In 1960, when France was on alert over the risk of terrorist attack by Algerian nationalists, Péchiney made its own security arrangements and organized its workers into armed foot patrols. Saint-Auban's unusual private status was not rescinded until the late 1980s.

This was the community into which Drummond blundered – a closed tribe that had learned to survive by looking after their own. In the blood-letting that followed the Liberation, two brothers living in Saint-Auban were shot on suspicion of collaborating with the Germans. It turned out to be a case of mistaken identity; the family were later sent a letter of apology by the head of the local Communist Party. No wonder so many people were convinced that the maquis held the key to unlocking the murder mystery – and no wonder the locals refused to co-operate with Sébeille during his investigation.

Jean-François was as convinced as I that the Drummonds' presence at La Grand'Terre in 1952 was no coincidence. The way the Hillman had been parked and many other details suggested a rendezvous to him, too, although he hadn't given much thought to whom the meeting might have been with.

'I think he was meeting someone from the factory,' I said, 'to gather information about what was going on here.'

'The factory? Here? But, why would Drummond care about Saint-Auban? I know he was a scientist but I thought his work was to do with food.'

I explained Drummond's secret war-work, his post-war position at Boots, his interest in chlorine technology, and the untested military potential of agrochemicals such as Lindane during the Cold War.

'Don't you think it's curious that the two most significant dates in Saint-Auban's Lindane production run, 1947 and 1952, were also the two years that Drummond was in the area?'

'He was here in 1947, too?'

'Maybe,' I said; and I launched into an account of the mysterious disappearance of the Long Eaton pocket diary.

'It's certainly possible,' Jean-François said when I had finished. 'What did you say Drummond's position at Boots was again?'

'Chef de Recherche.'

Jean-François emitted a low whistle. 'You're right. The . . . connections to this factory are very strange indeed.'

Another point had occurred to me – something that I had not thought of before Jean-François explained the relationship between Saint-Auban and the Rhône-Poulenc plant at Le Pont-de-Claix. On the third day of their five-day drive south towards Villefranche, the Drummonds stopped at Aix-les-Bains, a spa-town in the Rhône Alps. Domrémy, their previous stop, was Elizabeth's idea – she had wanted to see the birthplace of Joan of Arc – but no explanation was ever given for their visit to Aix-les-Bains. The choice had already struck me as strange. Aix-les-Bains was hardly a premier family tourist destination. Almost anywhere else would have been more fun for a ten-year-old girl than this quiet resort favoured by arthritic pensioners. Aix-les-Bains, moreover, was not really on the way to Villefranche from Domrémy. Why were they so anxious to spend a night there? Once again, the reason could have been innocent. On the other hand, Aix-les-Bains was less than 40 miles north of Le Pont-de-Claix. As with Villefranche, the distance from the putative target was convenient without looking suspicious: the perfect espionage-cum-holiday compromise.

Jean-François showed no sign of wanting to move from the car park where the HCH and Lindane sheds once stood. We sat together in silence for a minute or two, the factory tour temporarily forgotten, lost in mutual contemplation of the past. The car's engine ticked as it cooled.

'Did you know that Drummond's camera was never recovered from the Hillman?' I said eventually. 'My theory is that it was stolen because it contained photographs of Saint-Auban. Do you think that's possible?'

'It's perfectly possible. The factory was never a very secret kind of place. Look,' he said, twisting around in his seat.

I followed his finger. About 70 yards away and in direct line of sight was a pedestrian walkway attached to the side of a railway bridge.

'That's the old branch line to Digne. The bridge is disused now, but in the fifties the walkway was open to the public. People used it all the time to get across the river.'

'But it runs right through the middle of the plant!'

'Exactly. In fact, public access was only closed off quite recently.'

'And Drummond could have stood up there and taken photographs?'

'How could anyone have stopped him?'

He offered to show me the company archives, which were kept a short distance away at central headquarters. The building was another small gem of 1940s architecture. AFC, the initials of Alais Forges et Camargue, the firm that controlled the factory before Péchiney, were picked out in the ironwork of the staircase and repeated in modernist bas-relief across the cream-coloured façade. It took some time to get to the archives. Jean-François kept stopping to say hello to colleagues coming the other way, an elaborate Gallic ritual involving much banter and double-kisses all round. Finally I was led up to a disused boardroom under the eaves of the building. A layer of plaster dust covered everything, and the wall paint was peeling so badly that in one or two places it hung down in sheets like two-dimensional stalactites.

The company archive was actually a cupboard. Jean-François couldn't remember the last time anyone had opened it. Inside were seventeen grey cardboard box files that we took out and stacked in a low wall along the dirty boardroom table.

'Help yourself,' he said. 'I'll be in my office downstairs. Come and find me when you're finished.'

The boxes contained carbon copies of research notes dating back to the foundation of the factory. They were flimsy and yellowed with age; in some cases the ink-type had faded away altogether. Several had diagrams appended to them, hand-drawn in ink and meticulously annotated in copperplate. Chronologically arranged, the notes amounted to an extraordinary insight into the evolution of French chlorine technology over the twentieth century. I wasn't chemically literate enough to make proper sense of the material. Some of the recipes for weed-killers, like the one entitled *Fabrication d'un désherbant calcique à partir des liqueurs primaires chloruro-chloratées*, were little more than tongue-twisters to me. But it was evident that experiments on agrochemicals had formed a major part of the research laboratory's work over the years, and that these experiments had reached their apogee in the 1950s.

There were several papers on Lindane. One, an enquiry into the efficiency of the 'Thorp-Willermain' extraction method, was dated 1954 – which appeared to show that, two years into their production run, the Saint-Auban chemists had still not perfected the means by which Lindane was manufactured. This was just the sort of information that might have interested the Director of Research of a rival agrochemicals concern. Another research paper had a card stapled to it that forbade its circulation without permission from senior management. It was dated 1952.

'That's interesting,' Jean-François said when I showed him. 'It shows that management knew that at least some of its lab research was of actual or potential value to commercial rivals. I'm surprised – I didn't realize that what we were doing back then was so sensitive.'

'Could I . . . I don't suppose I could photocopy one or two of these?'

'Ooff! Take them if they're useful. No-one's interested in them any more. I'll give you something to put them in. Just promise to post them back when you're finished.'

And so it was that I left the factory carrying a courtesy Arkema shoulder-bag stuffed full of Cold War industrial secrets.

Melissa came with me on the final Drummonding expedition a few days later. We back-tracked through Saint-Auban once again, following the *Toutes Directions* signs until we found the N96. It was late afternoon, not far off the time of day (and time of year) that the Drummonds had taken the same fateful route.

'If you were looking for a place to camp, where would you stop?' I said as we bowled along. The N96 was a speedy road. Sections of it had recently been upgraded. Cars kept roaring up behind us, flashing their headlights impatiently and rocketing past wherever the bends in the road allowed it.

'We've passed plenty of places already. There was a turn-off a mile back that looked promising. Or – there,' Melissa pointed.

I slowed, stopped and reversed hastily back up the road with the hazard lights on for a better look, a manoeuvre that made Melissa screw her eyes tight shut and hide her head in her hands. We drove up another small turn-off for a hundred yards past an old stone-built farmhouse with horses in a paddock and chickens scratching in the dust. Next to it was a meadow filled with poppies and cornflowers that seemed to dance in the late afternoon sun. The road steepened to a bridge over an old irrigation canal bubbling with clean clear water.

'It's perfect,' said Melissa.

'And unchanged since the 1950s, wouldn't you say?'

'Since the 1850s, more like.'

As I knew from the decades of speculation about the milestone by the Hillman, La Grand'Terre was located precisely 6 kilometres beyond Peyruis. Our afternoon so far had been relaxed, but I felt oddly tense as we neared our goal, and our conversation dwindled. I was anxious not to overshoot the farm. It had also occurred to me that it might not exist any more – demolished, perhaps, with the widening of the N96.

I knew that La Grand'Terre had not been demolished immediately. Gaston instructed his daughter-in-law to sell it when he was convicted, after which it changed ownership several times. None of the new occupants was lucky. The first buyers turned it, ghoulishly, into a campsite. After that it became a petrol station, and then a pizzeria called La Montagnière, but by the 1990s it was derelict. It really wouldn't have been surprising to find there was nothing there any more, but in the end there was no mistaking the L-shaped farmhouse about which I had read so much. It was as close to the road as it was possible to be: there was barely room for a pedestrian to pass between the zooming traffic and the outside wall. The main building's downstairs windows were filled in with breeze blocks and looked in poor shape. The pink-washed outbuildings to the rear looked recently developed, however, while the cars parked in the courtyard indicated that the farm was now in business as a holiday hotel. A sign on a telegraph pole confirmed it: 'La Grand'Terre Gîtes,' it read. 'Locations Saisonnières'. Dominici tourism had evidently undergone a renaissance since the televised version of the Affair.

We pulled over onto a patch of gravel a couple of hundred yards from the house – the natural and most obvious place to stop on that stretch of fast road – and realized at once that we had done almost exactly as the Drummonds had, fifty-three years before. I got out of the car and stared, momentarily shocked by the feeling of familiarity. I had read so many accounts of the murders that I had unconsciously memorized the geography of this place. Here was the gravel track leading to the pretty stone railway bridge over which Elizabeth supposedly fled. There, across the road, was the culvert by which Jack's body was found, mysteriously covered by an upturned camp bed. And here, just by these trees, was where the Drummonds had parked their Hillman for the last time. Melissa looked at Amelia, asleep in the back of the car, and shivered.

I walked off to take a long-range photograph of the farmhouse. The orchard and alfalfa patch that once filled the intervening land had been replaced by a few rows of tomatoes and lettuces. The fecundity of this part of France was legendary, yet to my jaundiced eye even these simple vegetables seemed to be struggling. I was still framing my shot when a man came out of the house and waved at me with exaggerated slowness: he was obviously used to snoops. I waved back awkwardly, suddenly feeling foolish, and heard Melissa calling me back to the car in an urgent and melodramatic whisper. It wasn't the fact that we had been spotted that bothered her, however.

'Up there, across the road,' she murmured. 'Do you see anything?'

'What is it?'

'There was something moving.'

'Like a *sanglier*, you mean?'

'More like a person. It was sort of . . . drifting.'

I peered at the thick scrub on the slope that loomed above the culvert. There was an unusually long gap in the passing traffic so that the sultry air was suddenly filled with the sound of cicadas, but otherwise nothing and no-one moved.

'Wooo,' I said, but Melissa didn't smile.

'Please – can we not spend too long here?'

'OK, give me ten minutes.'

'Five.'

'OK.'

La Grand'Terre was a terrible misnomer. The farm wasn't *grand* but a narrow strip of wasteland, cut off from the world by the N96 on one side and a railway line on the other. The vegetation looked grimy; the edge of the property was dotted with cigarette butts, shreds of plastic and other swarf from the road. Even in the 1950s it must have been a wretched place to stop and camp. Back then it had at least been possible to cross over the railway via the bridge and follow the track down to the bank of the Durance, but now the bridge led nowhere. The path on the other side was blocked by a stout wire fence designed to separate wildlife from the travellers rushing along the new motorway immediately beyond it. The air was filled with the stereophonic drone of fast traffic.

I considered taking my shoes and socks off as I crossed the railway bridge. The soles of Elizabeth's feet had been examined by Dr Dragon, the first doctor to arrive at the murder scene, who noted that they were unblemished. His finding gave rise to later speculation that Elizabeth had not fled barefoot over this rough ground, as the police contended, but had been carried there either shortly before or immediately after her death. But the experiment felt somehow inappropriate – too disrespectful, too macabre – and I decided against it. It was the right decision, because just over the bridge I found a substantial shrine. The murder site had been transformed into a place of solemn remembrance.

There was no doubt as to which of the Drummonds the shrine was intended to commemorate. A makeshift cross was festooned with cuddly toys, their gaudy colours faded by the weather. There was a pink teddy and a yellow teddy, a green alligator in a waistcoat, a Bugs Bunny. There were flowers, too, most of them plastic but some of them real and fresh. I stopped to read a card pinned to the cellophane wrapped around a large and perfect red rose. 'Christelle Lungo –

Artisan Fleuriste,' it said; '9, cours Péchiney, Saint-Auban'. Rusty pots and other ornaments were heaped around the base of the cross in decaying layers. It was peculiar: Elizabeth had lived for only ten years, but it looked as though she had been mourned at this spot consistently for the last fifty-three. I found nothing specifically commemorating her parents. The French were sentimental in their grief: it had always been the murder of the innocent young girl that most pricked their collective conscience.

I followed the path as far as the deer-fence, where it branched left along the railway line and right back towards the farmhouse. Elizabeth's body had been found down and to the right by what was now the hard shoulder of the A51. I took the right-hand path for a short way, past a warning sign attached to a tree that depicted a man drowning: the outhouse where the Dominicis were supposed to have kept the Rock-Ola rifle had been torn down to make way for a swimming-pool. I disturbed a lizard in a small clearing, basking in the fading Provençal sunshine, and jumped as it scuttled away through the dry leaves. The undergrowth here had evidently been beaten back with weed-killer: a pile of empty plastic jerry cans had been dumped by a bush that had been spared. I turned one of them over with my foot for a closer look, wondering darkly if the blood that once poured out on this ground had been joined by the chemical that I was sure the Drummonds had died for. I wasn't wrong. The can had contained Dicuran, a herbicide made by Ciba-Geigy, the inventors of DDT. The chemical formula printed along the bottom revealed that it was indeed based on chlorine.

Melissa was calling from the car again to say that Amelia had woken up.

'Coming!' I shouted back.

I jiggled the jerry can with my foot. I was still thinking about the Drummonds and their horrible, violent end. I had spent a long time puzzling over who had killed them, and why – far longer than I'd ever expected to – yet I knew I was no nearer to solving the mystery, really, than when I started. Was Drummond on an intelligence-gathering mission related to the factory when he died? Despite all my probing, what little evidence I'd found to support the theory remained entirely circumstantial. In the end, my version of what happened was no better than anyone else's.

Did the Dominicis do it? It remained the likeliest solution. Not Gaston, perhaps, but Gustave and his scatter-brained nephew Roger Perrin, both of whom were drunk that night. In other words, the murders were random. Yet if I was sure of anything, it was that the Drummonds' presence at La Grand'Terre was not random. They were there, I still believed, for a secret rendez-vous with someone connected to the chlorine factory, and from whom Drummond hoped to collect sensitive industrial information.

Of the many possible permutations of what happened next, the one I preferred was this: the contact showed up eventually, only to discover that Drummond and his family were all dead. The imperative then was to remove and destroy anything that might link Drummond either to him or to the factory – hence the ransacked car and the missing camera. The Dominicis subsequently inculpated themselves, which was all to the good as it drew attention from the true reason that the Drummonds had been there.

This also suited the intelligence community in London, who later colluded in the cover-up by making sure that Drummond's pocket diary disappeared – together, perhaps, with the mysterious "documents" that Alain Dominici mentioned, missed in the dark by the ransacker, but found by the gendarmes in the light of day, only to be spirited away for ever via the British consulate in Marseilles. The English couple spoken to by Marquet, the traffic policeman in Digne, were not corporate assassins but secret service colleagues who were hurriedly pulled back to London when the murders were discovered – which would explain Sébeille's later failure to find or identify them.

The key to the mystery, as Alain Dominici realised, was Drummond's contact. Who might he have been? Father Lorenzi, the priest of

Ganagobie, seemed a strong possibility. He was pro-British, an ex-maquisard, a man of the cloth rather than a diehard Communist. He lived locally, and his flock had moved wholesale back to the factory floor when the war ended. He had the means and perhaps the motive to pass on secret information. At the very least, he would have made an excellent go-between. Yet there was no way I could prove it. The contact could equally have been any one of hundreds of factory workers – and it was pointless to pretend otherwise. Alain Dominici had spent a lifetime trying to untangle the knot. He lived almost in sight of the factory, and knew it and its workforce so well that he had once contemplated writing a history of the place. If he was stymied, what chance did I have? Standing there amongst the cleared undergrowth, the futility of my quest was apparent once again.

And yet I didn't feel as though I'd failed, somehow. It occurred to me that, ultimately, it didn't much matter who had killed the Drummonds, or why, because finding out would never put things right. Those terrible murders would always have happened, and the Drummonds were dust.

'James!' yelled Melissa.

The baby was mewling, the sound audible even above the noise of traffic. I hadn't been a father for long but I could recognize the demand for food when I heard it. Melissa was still breast-feeding, although there had been talk recently of switching to formula. I wasn't sure what to think about that. Which was better: bottle or breast? Thanks to the advent of chlorine technology, the problem was as insoluble as the murders. But at least Melissa and Amelia were alive. Unlike the Drummonds, they were the future.

'James!' Melissa yelled again.

I launched a kick at the jerry can at my feet. It flew through the air with a satisfying bop that made even the cicadas miss a beat. Then I turned and hurried back to the car, almost as anxious as Melissa was to be gone from this spooky place.

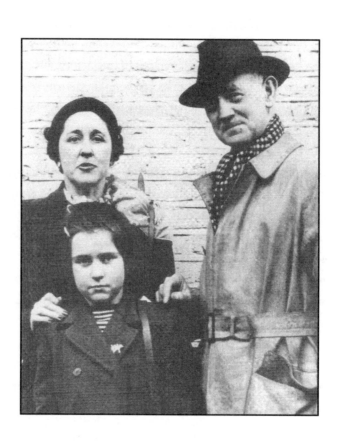

Postscript

Finding an infrared sauna in London wasn't easy. I rang my local gym, but they had never heard of infrared saunas. I tried Coco's Sunlounge and Massage Centre, the spa at the Berkeley Hotel, and even a gay pick-up joint in Covent Garden called the Sauna Bar, but none of them had heard of infrared either. Eventually I called the UK distributors of one of the best-selling infrared systems, a machine called a Physiotherm, who directed me to the Halo Wellbeing Centre: the only place in the whole of central London that carried their units, they said. I rang, was told that a forty-five-minute session would cost £20, and booked in Melissa and myself for the following day.

The Halo Centre was tucked down a quiet alley in Farringdon. It described itself in a brochure as 'an enclave of serenity amidst its frenetic urban surroundings'. The petite and nattily manicured receptionist spoke with a faint Californian accent.

'Take off your shoes and follow me,' she said.

Melissa gave me one of her looks, and I tried not to laugh. The receptionist led us along a corridor illuminated by tea-lights to a dim, windowless room in the basement where the walls were painted a cosmic orange. New age music, the formless, dreamy kind that I associated with West Country craft shops, tinkled from a small CD player. There was a table loaded with candles and little bottles of essential oils. Several books on Buddhist meditation techniques were arranged in a pile next to a futon on the floor. The Physiotherm, an enclosed wooden box with seating for two, hummed gently in the corner; blue light spilled through its glass door.

'Blue is associated with spiritual awareness,' purred the receptionist, 'but you can choose a different colour therapy if you want – violet, green, red or orange. Whatever you do, be sure to drink plenty of water.'

Then she left, and we stripped, giggling as we squeezed into the sauna. The experience might have been erotic, except that within ten minutes we were flinching uncomfortably in the energy that pulsed from the heater bars, and sweating as heavily as we had ever done in our lives.

'This,' said Melissa, 'is exactly like sitting in a microwave oven.'

'Don't worry,' I replied. 'It says here that there's no danger of actually cooking. Listen to this.'

With the help of a promotional pamphlet picked up at the entrance, I began to explain how the wavelength of the rays emanating from the machine was set to mimic the natural infrared heat generated by the human body.

'Thanks to something called resonant absorption,' I went on enthusiastically, 'fat molecules and clusters of contaminants in the body vibrate until they break up into particles small enough to pass out as sweat through the cell membranes . . .'

'James,' said Melissa.

'. . . Scientific analysis shows that infrared-induced sweat contains five to six times more toxins and impurities than normal sweat. Isn't this great? I'm sweltering.'

'James. Your nose is bleeding.'

I looked down to see that the salty torrent pouring from my body had indeed turned the most surprising shade of crimson.

'Quick,' I said, trying to staunch the flow with a pristine white towel, 'turn the light switch to red so that the blood doesn't show.'

'It says here on the instructions that red is associated with improved blood circulation.'

'Oh, shit. Green, then. Green is associated with healing.'

The lights started changing faster than in a cheap disco.

'If you started crying now,' Melissa giggled, 'We could tell people that getting rid of Lindane literally involves blood, sweat and tears.'

The nosebleed, a recurrence of an attack two days previously, wasn't the Physiotherm's fault and it didn't last long. The logic of infrared seemed perfectly sound. What bothered us more was the way it was presented. Scented candles and books on meditation were not exactly designed to appeal to the general population, while the assumption that Buddhists had some sort of monopoly over our well-being was frankly irritating. Sauna was a Finnish word, and the Physiotherm was made in Austria. Why wasn't the room outside painted Jägermeister green and decorated with antlers and Lederhosen? If sitting in an infrared sauna was the method of detoxification recommended by experts like John McLaren-Howard, it seemed strange that it was only available on the narcissistic fringes of alternative medical practice. Getting rid of toxins in the body was surely an obvious first step in the West's fight against cancer, not some half-baked hippy lifestyle choice. In a just world, infrared sauna sessions should have been available on the National Health Service.

After forty-five minutes the timer on the Physiotherm pinged to let us know that we were done. The litre bottle of Evian we had taken in with us had lasted all of twenty minutes, and I felt the light-headed beginnings of a headache that the relative cool of the scented room beyond did nothing to relieve. In the shower I scrubbed myself with a loofah until I tingled. It was a pleasant enough kind of purgatory, although Melissa was right when she said it shouldn't have been necessary in the first place. She was also right to ask how long one was supposed to persist with it. Was one session enough to decontaminate a body? Ten sessions? Once a week, perhaps? No-one, not McLaren-Howard and certainly not the Halo Centre's receptionist, was able to advise us. The only option was to go on with it for as long as we could, and then to resubmit ourselves to the attentions of Biolab to see if the treatment had worked – although I doubted whether Melissa would be amenable to that.

'Amelia is only going to eat organic food now that she's weaned,' she announced on the way home. 'I don't ever want her to have to go through this detox business.'

'Didn't you like the loofah I bought you?'

'No. It hurt my skin.'

'Oh. Well, in that case, organic lentils for Amelia it must be.'

In reality I knew that it would be impossible to control what our daughter ate in the future. As parents, the most we could achieve was to give her an early taste for proper food and hope that the preference lasted into adulthood. In the grand scheme of things, ensuring that what she consumed was free of potentially life-threatening chemicals was a secondary matter. But I still saw it as an important parental duty. The organic industry no longer felt faddish to either of us: it was simply common sense to shop for food on the precautionary principle. And while sitting in an infrared sauna was about trying to undo the agrochemical mistakes of the past, eating organic was about trying to ensure that those mistakes were not repeated, and so offered hope for the future.

There were some encouraging signs that the past complacency shown by government towards the risks of agrochemical farming was at last starting to crack. Not long after Melissa and I returned from France, Georgina Downs, the tireless anti-crop-spray campaigner from Runcton, scored a notable victory when the Royal Commission on Environmental Pollution agreed with her that the government had a case to answer, and recommended the introduction of a no-spray buffer zone around the edges of fields next to people's homes. It was the first time that a body of such seniority had admitted the possibility that the regulations governing crop-sprays were inadequate. The Commission acknowledged, too, that there was a plausible link between crop-sprays and statistical clusters around the country of diseases such as ME, Parkinson's and cancer.

She was loudly cheered for her achievement. One newspaper dubbed her 'Hurricane Georgina' for her uncompromising campaign style. Another compared her to Erin Brokovich, the real-life hero of the eponymous Julia Roberts film, who successfully sued a Californian power company in 1993 for damaging the health of hundreds of local residents with their hexavalent chromium pollution. Georgina later won a prestigious environmental award, leading *Farmers Weekly* to include her in their top twenty list of 'power players' in the British farming industry.

I rang to congratulate her after the Royal Commission report was published, only to discover that she was still far from satisfied. The no-spray buffer zone under proposal, I learned, was just 5 metres wide: a distance that she insisted was 'wholly inadequate'. When setting the width of the buffer zone, the Commission apparently relied on just one source: the government-funded Silsoe Research Institute, whose work related predominantly to crop-sprayer nozzle design and droplet drift. The SRI's expertise in spraydrift therefore extended only a short distance beyond the area treated. Their studies never took into account such pertinent factors as volatilization, or the effect of the prevailing wind. Yet in California, as Georgina pointed out, many commonly used crop-sprays had been detected as far as 50 miles from their site of application.

'The government has to start making the protection of public health its priority instead of simply protecting industry interests,' she commented.

I could see her point. A 5-metre buffer-zone wasn't going to do much to safeguard the public. The proposal was timid and smacked of reluctance – a token gesture born of research that was slapdash at best. Why did the Commission not seek further expert opinion before setting the buffer zone width? Incompetence? Or was it perhaps because 5 metres, really the shortest possible distance they could have come up with, suited the purposes of a body worried about the implications of a wider zone?

Whatever the reason, the feebleness of their recommendation strongly suggested that the whole mindset of the regulatory establishment was wrong. However much the system had been tightened up since the time of Williams and Zuckerman in the 1940s and 1950s, the old status quo between government and industry that underlay it was unchanged. In those days there was at least some social and military justification for the use of agrochemicals, but no-one in Europe was starving any more, and the military need for them disappeared when the Cold War ended. The only justification left was a commercial one.

It occurred to me that the regulators were operating a version of Gordon Hobday's therapeutic ratio: if the commercial advantages of a given agrochemical were deemed to outweigh the potential disadvantages – provided, most particularly, that it met 'acceptable' levels of pollution – then a licence could be granted for its use. But who was to say what an 'acceptable' level of pollution might be? It was certainly not acceptable to me that Melissa's breast milk contained traces of potential carcinogens. The Royal Commission thought that a crop-spray buffer zone of 5 metres was sufficient to protect public health in the future; research in California suggested that 50 miles might be required. With the facts so uncertain, would it not be wiser for the government to exercise the precautionary principle and to oblige industry to demonstrate the safety and necessity of their products – or else to withhold their licence? Put another way, why did the government not try to prevent pollution, instead of trying to manage it through regulation as it presently did? Georgina was right: it was the government's elected duty to protect the public's health, and it was wrong that the onus of proving a link between agrochemicals and disease still lay with the public after all these years.

The debate on public nutrition in Britain had shifted to the centre ground in the months since Melissa and I married. The growing frequency and sophistication of TV programmes and newspaper articles on the subject suggested that it had become a big media selling point – bigger, probably, than at any time since the 1940s. And as Drummond once appreciated, a better-educated public was a powerful thing. Nothing and no-one else could bring about cultural change so effectively. Jamie Oliver's *School Dinners* series was a case in point, causing such a stir that the government was finally forced to pledge an extra £220m towards better catering for schoolchildren; the TV chef later topped a Channel 4

News poll among viewers asked to name their most inspiring political figure of the year. Patrick Holden, the director of the Soil Association, even suggested in the *Daily Telegraph* that the public had reached what he called the 'tipping point . . . they don't want industrial farming. They know too much.'

It was certainly true that an increasing number of people distrusted industrial farming. Sales of organic food had risen by more than £100m a year in the last ten years. Three-quarters of people were worried about pesticide residues in foods, according to polls. Three-quarters of new British parents included organic food in their offspring's diet, and sales of organic milk had doubled in the past year. Yet the reason, it seemed to me, was not that the public knew too much, but that they understood too little. For all the hoop-la surrounding the organic movement, the evidence of its benefits remained circumstantial rather than proven. The decision to switch to organic was therefore not an informed choice but an intuitive one.

'We live in an evidence-based society where we cannot do anything until we have proof,' said Patrick Holden, 'but GM and BSE have taught us that you can have intuitive feelings about things that are against nature, that don't feel right. Good decisions, I believe, are made with a mixture of scientific and non-evidence-based criteria – including intuition.'

Holden obviously had a distinctive ecological agenda – he was an ex-farmer from a commune in Wales with a daughter called Barley – and I had seen for myself how easily intuition could be manipulated. But his words made a certain amount of sense, and Melissa and I could only do our best. Choosing organic would certainly remain the guiding principle by which we shopped for the foreseeable future. At the same time I was no longer quite as zealous about it as I once had been. I was conscious of the contradiction, but under Melissa's influence I had come to accept the necessity of compromise. In fact, keeping a sense of proportion about such things was the only way to stay sane. So if we were out at dinner with friends and salmon was served, I would now probably shut up and eat it; if we were at a restaurant, I would avoid the chicken but would otherwise order what I wanted without fussing too much about its provenance; if we were in a French market and Melissa said a home-grown pear was OK, I was ready to believe her. This certainly made for an easier life. Asceticism didn't suit either of us.

Besides, if I had learned anything it was that it was impossible to expunge all impurity from the chemicalized world that we lived in. Our future ingestion of chemicals would certainly be reduced by continuing to shop carefully for what we ate at home; our past contamination might also be reduced by exposing ourselves often enough to a bath of infrared energy. But nobody in the twenty-first century could hope to escape contamination altogether. The pollution of the earth had gone too far. Chemicals were not just in the food we ate but in the air that we breathed and the rain that fell on us, in the water we bathed in and the objects that we touched all the time in our everyday lives, and not even babies were born with a clean slate. That was the worst side-effect of the agrochemical revolution – sadder, by far, than the long-ago murder of a single English family in France. Perhaps the mother-to-child cycle of contamination will be broken one day. But for now, the agrochemical legacy of Drummond's generation remains the curse of ours.